Rehabilitation and Physical Therapy

Editors

DENIS J. MARCELLIN-LITTLE
DAVID LEVINE
DARRYL L. MILLIS

VETERINARY CLINICS OF NORTH AMERICA: SMALL ANIMAL PRACTICE

www.vetsmall.theclinics.com

January 2015 • Volume 45 • Number 1

ELSEVIER

1600 John F. Kennedy Boulevard • Suite 1800 • Philadelphia, Pennsylvania, 19103-2899
http://www.vetsmall.theclinics.com

**VETERINARY CLINICS OF NORTH AMERICA: SMALL ANIMAL PRACTICE Volume 45, Number 1
January 2015 ISSN 0195-5616, ISBN-13: 978-0-323-34188-2**

Editor: Patrick Manley
Developmental Editor: Susan Showalter

Veterinary Clinics of North America: Small Animal Practice (ISSN 0195-5616) is published bimonthly by Elsevier Inc., 360 Park Avenue South, New York, NY 10010-1710. Months of issue are January, March, May, July, September, and November. Business and Editorial Offices: 1600 John F. Kennedy Blvd., Ste. 1800, Philadelphia, PA 19103-2899. Customer Service Office: 3251 Riverport Lane, Maryland Heights, MO 63043. Periodicals postage paid at New York, NY and additional mailing offices. Subscription prices are $310.00 per year (domestic individuals), $500.00 per year (domestic institutions), $150.00 per year (domestic students/residents), $410.00 per year (Canadian individuals), $621.00 per year (Canadian institutions), $455.00 per year (international individuals), $621.00 per year (international institutions), and $220.00 per year (international and Canadian students/residents). To receive student/resident rate, orders must be accompanied by name of affiliated institution, date of term, and the *signature* of program/residency coordinator on institution letterhead. Orders will be billed at individual rate until proof of status is received. Foreign air speed delivery is included in all *Clinics* subscription prices. All prices are subject to change without notice. **POSTMASTER:** Send address changes to *Veterinary Clinics of North America: Small Animal Practice*, Elsevier Health Sciences Division, Subscription Customer Service, 3251 Riverport Lane, Maryland Heights, MO 63043. Customer Service (orders, claims, online, change of address): Elsevier Periodicals Customer Service, Elsevier Health Sciences Division Subscription Customer Service 3251 Riverport Lane Maryland Heights, MO 63043. Tel: 1-800-654-2452 (U.S. and Canada); 314-447-8871 (outside U.S. and Canada). Fax: 314-447-8029. E-mail: journalscustomerservice-usa@elsevier.com (for print support); journalsonlinesupport-usa@elsevier.com (for online support).

Reprints. For copies of 100 or more of articles in this publication, please contact the Commercial Reprints Department, Elsevier Inc., 360 Park Avenue South, New York, NY 10010-1710. Tel.: 212-633-3874; Fax: 212-633-3820; E-mail: reprints@elsevier.com.

Veterinary Clinics of North America: Small Animal Practice is also published in Japanese by Inter Zoo Publishing Co., Ltd., Aoyama Crystal-Bldg 5F, 3-5-12 Kitaaoyama, Minato-ku, Tokyo 107-0061, Japan.

Veterinary Clinics of North America: Small Animal Practice is covered in *Current Contents/Agriculture, Biology and Environmental Sciences, Science Citation Index, ASCA, MEDLINE/PubMed (Index Medicus), Excerpta Medica, and BIOSIS.*

Contributors

EDITORS

DENIS J. MARCELLIN-LITTLE
Diplome d'Etat de Docteur Veterinaire; Diplomate, American College of Veterinary Surgeons; Department of Clinical Sciences, College of Veterinary Medicine, North Carolina State University, Raleigh, North Carolina

DAVID LEVINE, PT, PhD, DPT, CCRP, Cert. DN
Diplomate, American Board of Physical Therapy Specialties (Orthopedics); Professor and Walter M. Cline Chair of Excellence in Physical Therapy, Department of Physical Therapy, University of Tennessee at Chattanooga, Chattanooga, Tennessee

DARRYL L. MILLIS, MS, DVM, CCRP
Diplomate, American College of Veterinary Surgeons; Diplomate, American College of Veterinary Sports Medicine and Rehabilitation; Department of Small Animal Clinical Sciences, College of Veterinary Medicine, University of Tennessee, Knoxville, Tennessee

AUTHORS

BARBARA BOCKSTAHLER, Dr.med.vet, DVM, PD, CCRP
Department für Kleintiere und Pferde, University of Veterinary Medicine, Vienna, Austria

IONUT ALEXANDRU CIUPERCA, DVM, MSc, CCRP
Department of Small Animal Clinical Sciences, College of Veterinary Medicine, University of Tennessee, Knoxville, Tennessee; VetPhysioCenter Bucuresti, Bucharest, Romania

MICHAEL S. DAVIS, DVM, PhD
Department of Physiological Sciences, Center for Veterinary Health Sciences, Oklahoma State University, Stillwater, Oklahoma

NANCY D. DOYLE, MPT
Gulf Coast Veterinary Specialists, Houston, Texas

MARTI G. DRUM, DVM, PhD
Department of Small Animal Clinical Sciences, College of Veterinary Medicine, University of Tennessee, Knoxville, Tennessee

JUNE HANKS, PT, PhD, DPT, CWS, CLT
Department of Physical Therapy, University of Tennessee at Chattanooga, Chattanooga, Tennessee

MAJ ANDREA L. HENDERSON, DVM, CCRP
Chief, Rehabilitation, Department of Defense Military Working Dog Veterinary Service; Joint Base San Antonio - Lackland, San Antonio, Texas

CHRISTIAN LATIMER, DVM
Department of Small Animal Clinical Sciences, College of Veterinary Medicine, University of Tennessee, Knoxville, Tennessee

DAVID LEVINE, PT, PhD, DPT, CCRP, Cert. DN
Diplomate, American Board of Physical Therapy Specialties (Orthopedics); Professor and
Walter M. Cline Chair of Excellence in Physical Therapy, Department of Physical Therapy,
University of Tennessee at Chattanooga, Chattanooga, Tennessee

DENIS J. MARCELLIN-LITTLE
Diplome d'Etat de Docteur Veterinaire; Diplomate, American College of Veterinary
Surgeons; Department of Clinical Sciences, College of Veterinary Medicine,
North Carolina State University, Raleigh, North Carolina

SUSAN S. McDONALD, EdD, OTR/L
Department of Occupational Therapy, Chattanooga, Tennessee

DARRYL L. MILLIS, MS, DVM, CCRP
Diplomate, American College of Veterinary Surgeons; Diplomate, American College of
Veterinary Sports Medicine and Rehabilitation; Department of Small Animal Clinical
Sciences, College of Veterinary Medicine, University of Tennessee, Knoxville, Tennessee

BRIAN PRYOR, PhD
LiteCure LLC, Newark, Delaware

JOANNA FREEMAN PYKE, PT, BSc.KINE
Private Practice, Oakville, Ontario, Canada

CORY SIMS, DVM
Department of Clinical Sciences, College of Veterinary Medicine, North Carolina State
University, Raleigh, North Carolina

RENNIE WALDRON, DVM
Department of Clinical Sciences, College of Veterinary Medicine, North Carolina State
University, Raleigh, North Carolina

Contents

This article reviews some important studies regarding canine physical rehabilitation. Bones, cartilage, muscles, ligaments, and tendons undergo atrophy if loading is decreased. Knowledge of the changes that occur with immobilization and the time course of events helps in the development of a rehabilitation program to improve tissue integrity. Outcome assessment instruments are clinically useful indicators of patient progress and the success of rehabilitation programs. A number of physical modalities are used in canine rehabilitation, although there are relatively few canine-specific studies. Rehabilitation has specific benefits in the treatment of various orthopedic and neurologic conditions.

Physical agent modalities can be effective components of the overall rehabilitation of small animals. This article reviews the effects, indications, contraindications, and precautions of cold, superficial heat, therapeutic ultrasound, and electrical stimulation.

Laser therapy is an increasingly studied modality that can be a valuable tool for veterinary practitioners. Mechanisms of action have been studied and identified for the reduction of pain and inflammation and healing of tissue. Understanding the basics of light penetration into tissue allows evaluation of the correct dosage to deliver for the appropriate condition, and for a particular patient based on physical properties. New applications are being studied for some of the most challenging health conditions and this field will continue to grow. Additional clinical studies are still needed and collaboration is encouraged for all practitioners using this technology.

Optimal function after injury, surgery, or in patients with chronic conditions requires adequate motion in joints, muscles, tendon, fascia, and skin. Range of motion and stretching exercises are commonly used in companion animal rehabilitation programs to maintain or improve motion of musculoskeletal tissues. Range of motion exercises and stretching prevent adhesions from forming, help scar tissue remodeling, may improve muscle tone, and prevent future injury from occurring. Stretching is used to avoid loss of motion or to regain lost joint motion. Stretching is done manually, using external coaptation, or using therapeutic exercises. Careful documentation of range of motion is necessary.

Therapeutic exercises are the cornerstone of the rehabilitation programs of companion animals. Therapeutic exercises are used to improve active joint range of motion, to improve weight bearing and limb use, to build strength and muscle mass, and to increase conditioning (eg, endurance, speed). Each case is unique as chronicity, type of injury, patient signalment and temperament, owner compliance, and level of required functional recovery vary widely. Therapeutic exercises are also essential for partial return to work or performance and to learn to perform activities of daily living after injury or surgery.

A specific diagnosis is needed to perform optimal rehabilitation of orthopedic problems. A well-planned rehabilitation program is important for orthopedic patients when surgical repairs are mechanically weak (eg, when repairing fractures in skeletally immature patients or when repairing tendons or ligaments). Joint immobilization is sometimes used to protect weak surgical repairs. The duration of immobilization should be minimized, particularly in situations with potential loss of joint motion. Evidence-based information regarding specific modalities and techniques for rehabilitation of injured dogs and cats is limited. The choice of modalities and techniques must be based on common sense, knowledge of rehabilitation techniques, and clinical experience.

A comprehensive physiotherapy plan for neurology patients manages pain, prevents secondary complications, and supports the health and function of musculoskeletal tissues during recovery. Neurologically impaired patients range in ability from complete immobility (tetraplegia/paraplegia), partial mobility (tetraparesis/paraparesis), mild ataxia, to pain only. Important considerations for the design of a physiotherapy program include access to the patient, level of staff support, and safety of staff, patient, and client during treatments. A thorough overview of the treatment plan and expected outcome should be discussed with the client at the onset of therapy and should be reviewed frequently, particularly as the patient's status changes.

Patients who have total joint arthroplasty have varying needs related to rehabilitation. In the short term, rehabilitation should be used in all dogs to identify high-risk patients and to minimize the likelihood of postoperative complications. Many patients undergoing total hip replacement recover uneventfully without needing long-term physiotherapy. All patients undergoing total knee replacement and total elbow replacement need rehabilitation to restore limb use and maximize their functional recovery. This article presents rehabilitation considerations for companion animals undergoing total hip replacement, total knee replacement, and total elbow replacement; postoperative complications and how to mitigate risks; and anticipated patient outcomes.

Orthoses and Exoprostheses for Companion Animals

Denis J. Marcellin-Little, Marti G. Drum, David Levine, and Susan S. McDonald

Exoprostheses are devices that are secured to incomplete limbs to enable locomotion. By comparison, orthoses are devices externally applied to support or protect an injured body part. Orthoses also can be used to control, guide, protect, limit motion of, or immobilize an extremity, a joint, or a body segment. Exoprostheses and orthoses are a growing aspect of the physical rehabilitation of companion animals. They require precise design and fabrication. Patients and owners must be trained to use the devices. Exoprostheses and orthoses can have a profound beneficial impact on the mobility and the quality of life of companion animals.

Feline Rehabilitation

Marti G. Drum, Barbara Bockstahler, David Levine, and Denis J. Marcellin-Little

Cats have orthopedic problems, including osteoarthritis, fractures, and luxations that are positively impacted by physical rehabilitation. Most cats have an independent behavior that requires using a tactful approach to rehabilitation. Cats often do well with manual therapy and electrophysical modalities. Feline rehabilitation sessions may be shorter than canine rehabilitation sessions. Cats do best with therapeutic exercises when these exercises are linked to hunting, playing, or feeding.

VETERINARY CLINICS OF NORTH AMERICA: SMALL ANIMAL PRACTICE

RELATED INTEREST

Veterinary Clinics of North America: Exotic Animal Practice
January 2011, Volume 14, Issue 1
Analgesia and Pain Management
Joanne Paul-Murphy, *Editor*

THE CLINICS ARE NOW AVAILABLE ONLINE!
Access your subscription at:
www.theclinics.com

Preface

Veterinary Rehabilitation and Physical Therapy

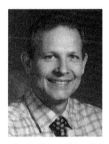
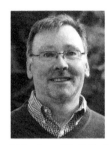
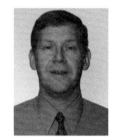

Denis J. Marcellin-Little, DEDV

David Levine, PT, PhD, DPT, CCRP, Cert. DN

Darryl L. Millis, MS, DVM, DACVS, CCRP, DACVSMR

Editors

It has been 10 years since *Veterinary Clinics of North America: Small Animal Practice* dedicated an issue to rehabilitation and physical therapy. During that period of time, the field has been growing steadily, and the American College of Veterinary Sports Medicine and Rehabilitation has been established. It is time to share new developments and techniques that are used in the rehabilitation of companion animals. The same group of editors who collaborated on the 2005 issue has been collaborating on the current issue, and an outstanding group of authors has joined the editors to prepare the content.

This issue of *Veterinary Clinics of North America: Small Animal Practice* contains 10 articles that present new and updated general information on the scientific foundation of rehabilitation, therapeutic modalities, therapeutic exercise, and nutrition for patients undergoing rehabilitation. The use of therapeutic lasers has grown in recent years, and an article is dedicated to this emerging therapy. Two articles cover physical activities, focusing on stretching and range of motion and on therapeutic exercises. Several articles focus on patients with specific problems: orthopedic patients, neurologic patients, patients in need of orthosis and exoprostheses, and sporting dogs. For the first time in the veterinary literature, an article is dedicated to the needs of dogs and cats recovering from total joint arthroplasty. Another article focuses on cats undergoing rehabilitation.

The information included in this issue is intended to be readily applied to the practice of rehabilitation and physical therapy. Many patients still experience slow recoveries and complications that could potentially be avoided if practical and cost-effective rehabilitation programs were included. Nevertheless, the field has experienced considerable growth over the last 10 years. Rather than being an exotic and alternative form of practice, physical rehabilitation is now an integral part of practice for many clinicians who help patients recover from injuries and surgery.

Vet Clin Small Anim 45 (2015) ix–x
http://dx.doi.org/10.1016/j.cvsm.2014.10.001
0195-5616/15/$ – see front matter © 2015 Published by Elsevier Inc.

The editors sincerely hope that the information included in this issue positively impacts the practice of rehabilitation and the lives of injured companion animals and their owners.

Denis J. Marcellin-Little, DEDV
Department of Clinical Sciences
College of Veterinary Medicine
North Carolina State University
1052 William Moore Drive
Raleigh, NC 27607, USA

David Levine, PT, PhD, DPT, CCRP, Cert. DN
Department of Physical Therapy
University of Tennessee at Chattanooga
615 McCallie Avenue
Chattanooga, TN 37403, USA

Darryl L. Millis, MS, DVM, DACVS, CCRP, DACVSMR
Department of Small Animal Clinical Sciences
College of Veterinary Medicine
University of Tennessee
2407 River Drive
Knoxville, TN 37996, USA

E-mail addresses:
denis_marcellin@ncsu.edu (D.J. Marcellin-Little)
David-Levine@utc.edu (D. Levine)
dmillis@utk.edu (D.L. Millis)

Evidence for Canine Rehabilitation and Physical Therapy

Darryl L. Millis, MS, DVM, DACVS, CCRP, DACVSMR[a],*,
Ionut Alexandru Ciuperca, DVM, MSc, CCRP[a,b]

KEYWORDS

- Canine rehabilitation • Physical Therapy • Evidence-based medicine
- Musculoskeletal tissue disuse • Outcome assessment
- Therapeutic and aquatic exercises • Physical modalities
- Orthopedic rehabilitation • Neurologic rehabilitation

KEY POINTS

- Cartilage, muscle, tendons, ligaments, and bone undergo atrophy with decreased limb use. Appropriate rehabilitation of musculoskeletal conditions must incorporate this knowledge to safely remobilize and strengthen these tissues.
- The ideal outcome assessment instrument should be objective, easy to apply, inexpensive, noninvasive, and, most important, able to discriminate the effectiveness of treatments.
- Therapeutic and aquatic exercises, heat, cold, therapeutic ultrasound, electrical stimulation, therapeutic laser, extracorporeal shock wave, and pulsed electromagnetic fields have all been used in veterinary rehabilitation and have benefit.
- Research indicates that rehabilitation is useful for the treatment of various orthopedic and neurologic conditions.

Rehabilitation and physical therapy of companion animals are among the fastest growing branches of veterinary medicine. The scientific evidence regarding the efficacy of canine rehabilitation and physical therapy is relatively small, but that body of literature is growing. Twenty years ago, there was scant anecdotal information regarding rehabilitation in animals, and in particular, dogs. Most of the early literature pertaining to canine rehabilitation was based on the dog as a model for physical therapy in people. This information is important, yet it is often found in journals related to human physical therapy, and exercise and sport science. Fortunately, the advent of computer-based databases has increased the accessibility of these sources. Others

[a] Department of Small Animal Clinical Sciences, College of Veterinary Medicine, University of Tennessee, 2407 River Drive, Knoxville, TN 37996, USA; [b] VetPhysioCenter Bucuresti, 25 Virgil Plesoianu Street, Bucharest, Romania
* Corresponding author.
E-mail address: dmillis@utk.edu

have extrapolated information determined in human beings undergoing physical therapy, but these results may or may not apply to animals. Yet, it may be the best available information. Today, there is growing interest in answering not only the question, "Does it work?", but also "How does it work?", and "How much benefit is there?" Importantly, there is growing interest among surgeons, internists, neurologists, and members of the newly formed American College of Veterinary Sports Medicine and Rehabilitation. Clinicians involved with rehabilitation are challenged to ask questions related to canine rehabilitation and physical therapy, but more important, to find the answers through new research.

RESPONSES OF TISSUES TO DISUSE AND REMOBILIZATION

The responses of musculoskeletal tissues to disuse and remobilization in dogs and other animals have been reviewed.[1] This article reviews some of the important studies regarding dogs. It is obvious that if bones, cartilage, muscles, ligaments, and tendons are not loaded and used, atrophy occurs. The more important questions are "How much atrophy occurs?", and "Over what time frame do atrophic changes occur?" Equally important are the questions, "How can tissues be safely remobilized and strengthened" and "How long will it take to regain the lost tissue integrity?"

Cartilage

Chondrocytes, proteoglycans, collagen, and water are the main components of articular cartilage, and each plays a unique role in maintaining the structure and function of cartilage. With disuse or immobilization of joints, there is cartilage atrophy and thinning of articular cartilage, decreased synovial fluid production and distribution, diminished delivery of oxygen and nutrients to cartilage, reduced proteoglycan content and synthesis, and decreased cartilage stiffness. For example, 3 to 11 weeks of immobilization of a stifle joint in flexion results in 13% to 60% reduction of proteoglycan content in young dogs, and cartilage thickness may be reduced 9% to 50%.[2,3] In addition, the method of joint immobilization affects cartilage. If joints are immobilized in flexion without weight bearing, cartilage atrophy occurs. Conversely, if joints are immobilized in extension and weight bearing is allowed, the joint may undergo degenerative changes. In any case, joint immobilization is not desirable. However, there are clinical situations that require joint immobilization. Knowledge of the changes that occur with immobilization and the time course of events helps in the development of a rehabilitation program to improve tissue integrity.

The length of immobilization, condition of cartilage, and the length and magnitude of weight bearing after immobilization affect cartilage recovery. After 6 weeks of immobilization, 3 weeks of free, low-intensity activity resulted in normal cartilage in 1 study.[4] Longer periods of immobilization likely require longer recovery times. For example, immobilization for longer than 15 weeks may not result in complete recovery, even with 50 weeks of remobilization, in young dogs.[5] Vigorous exercise after immobilization may be deleterious to cartilage. In 1 study, jogging young dogs 9.5 km/d at 5 km/h after immobilization for 3 weeks resulted in continued decreases in cartilage thickness (20%) and proteoglycan content (35%), even though proteoglycan synthesis increased (16%).[6]

Bone

Situations that prevent or reduce weight bearing on a limb result in reduced cortical and cancellous bone mass, cortical bone density and stiffness, and increased turnover in cancellous bone.[7,8] The changes that occur after immobilization vary depending on the length of immobilization, age of the animal, and the bone involved. The effects seem to be more profound in younger dogs. In fact, immature dogs demonstrated a 55% decrease in bone mass of the distal tibial metaphysis after 4 weeks of unilateral hindlimb cast immobilization in 1 study.[9] Trabecular bone is affected to a greater degree than cortical bone, and the effects of immobilization are more extensive in the more distal weight-bearing bones.[10,11] Biomechanical properties of cortical and cancellous bone are also significantly affected by immobilization. Forelimbs of dogs immobilized for 16 weeks had decreased cortical load, yield, and stiffness as well as cancellous bone failure stress, yield stress, and modulus, compared with control limbs.[12] In general, immobilized limb cancellous bone mechanical properties were 28% to 74% of control values, and cortical bone mechanical properties were 71% to 98% of control values.

Like cartilage, bone has the capacity to regain mass and biomechanical properties with remobilization. The potential for recovery of bone lost during disuse, both in the diaphyseal cortical and metaphyseal cancellous bone, was evaluated in young adult and old beagle dogs.[13] After immobilization of a forelimb for up to 32 weeks, there was considerable recovery of the original bone loss during remobilization. In both age groups, the residual deficits increased with the duration of immobilization and were similar in the metaphysis and in the diaphysis. In addition, the distal, weight-bearing bones tended to show greater losses and also greater recovery of bone. Older dogs had greater residual deficits, most evident in the diaphysis. After 32 weeks of immobilization and 28 weeks of remobilization, a 50% loss in the third metacarpal diaphysis of younger dogs immediately after the immobilization period decreased to 15% (a 70% recovery), whereas older dogs had a 38% loss that decreased to 23% (a 40% recovery). In contrast, immobilization for 6 or 12 weeks resulted in complete recovery of bone after remobilization of 10 or 28 weeks, respectively. Mild treadmill activity after free remobilization may also be beneficial for dogs with immobilized limbs. Forelimb immobilization of 1- to 2-year-old dogs for 16 weeks, followed by a remobilization period of 16 weeks of kennel confinement and 16 weeks of treadmill exercise administered 3 times per week, resulted in the return of cortical and cancellous bone mineral density and mechanical properties to essentially normal levels.[12]

Muscle

Muscles are perhaps the most obvious musculoskeletal tissues that are recognized to undergo atrophy during periods of immobilization and disuse. Unlike bone, cartilage, ligaments or tendons, changes in muscle mass may be evident in dogs with limb injuries or during postoperative recovery by palpation or observation in severe cases of muscle atrophy. The muscles most vulnerable to disuse atrophy are the postural muscles that contain a relatively large proportion of type I (slow-twitch) muscle fibers, extensor muscles, and muscles that cross a single joint.[14,15] Muscle strength decreases rapidly during the first week of immobilization, with further losses occurring more gradually over time.[16] The change in muscle fiber size and fiber percentage was studied in dog quadriceps muscles after 10 weeks of rigid immobilization.[15] Muscle fiber atrophy was greatest in the vastus medialis and least in the rectus femoris. Atrophy of type I fibers was, in order from most to least atrophied, vastus medialis, vastus lateralis, and rectus femoris; for type II fibers, atrophy of the vastus medialis was equal to vastus lateralis, and both atrophied more than the rectus femoris. Vastus medialis types I and II muscle fiber areas were only about one third of normal after immobilization. A similar study with 10 weeks of immobilization indicated that there was a significant decrease in both types I and II fiber areas, and muscle fiber areas recovered to only approximately 70% of control values after 4 weeks of remobilization.[17]

Changes in muscle mass are common in dogs with cranial cruciate ligament rupture, and after surgical treatment of the injury. In an experimental study, dogs had a cranial cruciate ligament transected, followed by immediate stabilization with an extracapsular procedure.[18] Results of this study revealed muscle atrophy of the surgical leg by 2 weeks, with muscle mass beginning to return between 4 and 8 weeks; significant atrophy was still present 8 weeks after surgery. In addition, the contralateral nonsurgical limb underwent hypertrophy, possibly because of the increased loading on that limb during recovery. A study of dogs with naturally occurring cranial cruciate ligament deficiency evaluated patients before surgical treatment and 1.5, 7, and 13 months after surgery.[19] The degree of quadriceps muscle atrophy present before surgery correlated significantly with the degree of cartilage fibrillation, indicating a relationship with the severity of the condition. Although there was slightly greater muscle atrophy 6 weeks after surgery, muscle mass improved 7 and 13 months after surgery, although significant residual muscle atrophy remained in many dogs even after 1 year. A measure of quadriceps atrophy may be a useful tool for assessing long-term outcome.

The clinical aspects and biochemical changes in dogs with induced muscle atrophy followed by various levels of physical rehabilitation were studied.[20] Muscle atrophy was induced by joint immobilization for 30 days. Groups included (1) control, (2) massage, passive range of motion, and neuromuscular electrical stimulation (NMES), (3) massage, passive range of motion and aquatic therapy in underwater treadmill, and (4) massage, passive range of motion, NMES, and aquatic therapy on an underwater treadmill. Degree of lameness, range of motion, thigh circumference, and serum creatine kinase and lactate dehydrogenase levels were measured. The authors concluded that therapeutic modalities such as massage, passive range of motion, NMES, and underwater treadmill walking accelerate clinical recovery in dogs with induced muscle atrophy.

Tendons and Ligaments

As with other musculoskeletal tissues previously discussed, tendons and ligaments undergo changes with disuse and immobilization. In many cases of tendon or ligament injury, a period of immobilization is necessary to prevent catastrophic failure of the affected structure(s). However, there is an adverse decline in structural and material properties of ligaments and tendons with immobilization of the joints that they cross. Even if some joint motion is allowed, stress deprivation rapidly reduces the mechanical properties of the tendon and ligament tissues.[21] The bone–tendon/bone–ligament complex is especially affected by immobilization.

In general, the cross-sectional area of the ligament or tendon is reduced; the parallel structure of fibrils and cells is disorganized; collagen turnover, synthesis, and degradation are increased with a net decrease in collagen mass; and glycosaminoglycan, hyaluronic acid, chondroitin sulfate, dermatan sulfate, and water content are decreased.[21] Remobilization returns the mechanical properties to near normal over time, but the recovery of the bony insertion sites is prolonged compared with the ligament–tendon mid substance. The effect of immobilization on the cranial cruciate ligament of dogs was studied using a model of internal skeletal fixation for 12 weeks.[22] The femur–ligament–tibia complex failed at the tibial insertion of the ligament for both experimental and control limbs. However, the load at failure and stiffness of the immobilized limbs were 45% and 73%, respectively, of the nonimmobilized cranial cruciate ligament. The loss of collagen was greater in the tibia and femur than in the cranial cruciate ligament, and correlated with mechanical failure at the bone insertion. The importance of bone resorption owing to disuse and its relationship to strength of the medial collateral and cranial cruciate ligament complexes was also evaluated in a cast immobilization study. Changes in the tibial insertion of the ligament were apparent, including the presence of osteoclasts, large fibroblasts, and replacement of bone by loosely arranged fibrous tissue.[23] Restriction of activity to cage confinement also causes significant bone atrophy of the tibial insertion sites of the collateral ligaments if adequate activity is not allowed. Additionally, there is decreased thickness of ligament and tendon fiber bundles, greater extensibility per unit load, and unchanged collagen content after immobilization.[24]

Although the mechanical properties of immobilized ligaments return to normal relatively quickly, the load to failure of the bone–ligament–bone complex lag behind, indicating that there is asynchronous healing of the bone–ligament–bone complex.[21] After 6 weeks of immobilization of the lower limbs of dogs, 18 weeks of remobilization was necessary for return of the normal structural properties of the medial femoral–tibial ligament complex.[23] In fact, up to 1 year of remobilization may be required for normalization of the ligament–tibia complex in some instances, whereas the mechanical properties of the ligament return to normal in a relatively short period of time, as newly synthesized collagen fibers gradually mature and strengthen with subsequent stress resumption of activity. Maintaining some joint motion and reducing the period of immobilization may help to preserve ligament and tendon properties. The article regarding rehabilitation of selected orthopedic conditions by Henderson et al in this edition provides additional details regarding these principles.

OUTCOME ASSESSMENT

Before determining whether or not a particular rehabilitation program has positive effects on a group of patients, adequate outcome assessment tools must be available to measure the response(s) to treatment(s). The ideal outcome assessment instrument should be objective, easy to apply, inexpensive, noninvasive, and most important, able to discriminate the effectiveness of treatments.

Activities of Daily Living and Return to Function

Activities of daily living and return to function are perhaps the most clinically useful indicators of the success of rehabilitation programs. Neurologic patients may be evaluated regarding the ability to complete certain tasks, such as changing body position without assistance, maintain a standing position for a given time, walk without falling or stumbling, and performing activities such as going up several steps or negotiating Cavaletti rails. Recent technology has made measurement of activity in the home environment relatively accessible and inexpensive. Pedometers, accelerometers, and global positioning system (GPS) devices worn by dogs give an absolute or relative indication of the amount of activity dogs have in their home environment.[25] These measurements may be important in obese dogs undergoing weight loss, or arthritic dogs that have decreased activity. Some devices have the ability to send a report to the owner by Wi-Fi or Bluetooth to a smart phone or computer.

The effectiveness of rehabilitation programs in working or sporting dogs is perhaps more easily measured by performance on the job or during an event. For example, the time achieved by a dog competing in flyball is relatively easy to measure. Other sports that have different obstacles and distances for each competition, such as agility and lure coursing, may not be measured as reliably with a particular time, but their relative performance against common competitors and the level of competition are reasonable indicators. Some working dogs, such as police dogs, may not be able to return to vigorous duties such as apprehension work, but they may be able to return to explosive and narcotic detection duties.

A 6-minute walk test determines the distance that an animal can walk in 6 minutes, and has been evaluated in healthy dogs and dogs with pulmonary disease.[26] The 6-minute walk test is used in human medicine to assess impairment, and to provide an objective measurement of disease progression and response to therapy. Healthy dogs walked 522.7 ± 52.4 m, whereas dogs with pulmonary conditions walked 384.8 ± 41.0 m. The authors concluded that the 6-minute walk test was easy to perform and discriminated between healthy dogs and dogs with pulmonary disease. However, further studies in dogs with other conditions are needed. In particular, the distance walked depends on the handler, the motivation of the dog, and the speed of the handler.

Gait Analysis

Gait may be analyzed subjectively or objectively, with pros and cons of each. Subjective analysis is relatively quick, inexpensive, and does not require equipment. Experience is important, but even seasoned gait evaluators may have difficulty characterizing gait abnormalities, especially if several joints or limbs are involved. In general, our eyes focus on the most obvious abnormality or factor contributing to gait asymmetry. However, multiple areas are affected frequently, including the spine. In addition, the sensitivity of subjective gait analysis is less compared with objective methods of gait evaluation. Conversely, objective gait measures, such as force platform or pressure walkways, generally assess only walking and trotting. Evaluation of activities such as ascending and descending stairs or stepping over obstacles may be difficult with objective gait analysis, but are readily evaluated subjectively. In fact, some dogs with relatively normal gait assessment by force platform analysis may have difficulty negotiating stairs.

Again, technology has made subjective gait analysis somewhat easier. Watching dogs walking and trotting on a treadmill may allow a more consistent gait pattern with minimal distractions. Also, the evaluator is able to watch a specific limb, joint, or footfall pattern repeatedly without moving or changing their focal distance. Filming dogs and assessing gait in slow motion allows observation of subtle gait abnormalities that may not be detected at real-time speed. Several software applications have become available to evaluate joint motion relatively inexpensively, but the accuracy of these programs must be validated and compared with traditional gait analysis techniques. Recording the gait of dogs is advised to compare changes over time because the ability to recall previous gait evaluations may be difficult, and subjective scoring systems may not distinguish subtle changes.

Weight bearing at a stance may be performed with computerized systems[27] or with simple systems, such as bathroom scales. Hyytiainen and coworkers[28] assessed the asymmetry of hind limbs of dogs with osteoarthritis (OA) by using a force platform during gait and in static weight bearing by using bathroom scales. The sensitivity of static weight-bearing measurements using bathroom scales was 39%, and specificity was 85%. The authors concluded that bathroom scales are a reliable, simple, cost-effective, and objective method for measuring static weight bearing and can be used as an outcome measure when rehabilitating dogs with osteoarthritic changes in the hind limbs.

Objective gait analysis has documented normal forces (kinetic gait analysis), and joint motion and stride length (kinematic gait analysis) during walking and trotting (**Figs. 1** and **2**).[29–31] In addition, several studies have evaluated gait in dogs with

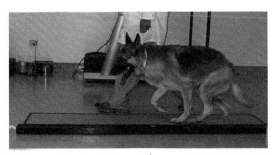

Fig. 1. A 1-year-old German shepherd dog with a partially amputated right hind limb is walking on a pressure-sensitive walkway for objective assessment of his weight distribution before receiving a prosthetic foot. (*Photograph courtesy of* D Marcellin-Little.)

various musculoskeletal abnormalities or neurologic conditions, including hip dysplasia, elbow arthritis, and cranial cruciate ligament rupture.[32–36] Most studies have shown compensatory changes in joints and limbs as a result of a primary problem. Further, a technique known as inverse dynamics combines kinetic and kinematic gait analysis and estimates muscle moments surrounding the joints.[37–39]

Joint Motion

Joint motion has traditionally been measured with a goniometer (**Fig. 3**). The normal joint motion of Labrador retriever dogs and cats has been established.[40,41] There is good correlation with goniometric measurements made from radiographs at maximum joint flexion and extension angles. In addition, different evaluators may obtain similar measurements when appropriate bony landmarks are used. Goniometry has been used to evaluate stifle range of motion in dogs with cranial cruciate ligament insufficiency. There seems to be an association with lameness and stifle extension after stifle stabilization surgery.

Additional information is needed regarding goniometry of different breeds and body types. Also, information regarding goniometry of various conditions and the response to rehabilitation is lacking. Furthermore, joint flexion and extension angles are commonly measured, but other accessory joint motions have not been adequately

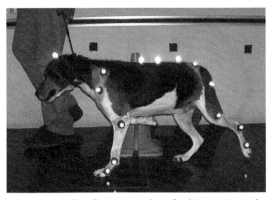

Fig. 2. A dog is instrumented with reflective markers for kinematic evaluation of gait. (*From* Millis DL, Levine D. Assessing and measuring outcomes. In: Millis DL, Levine D, editors. Canine rehabilitation and physical therapy. St Louis (MO): Saunders; 2014. p. 224; with permission.)

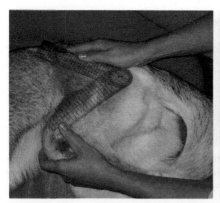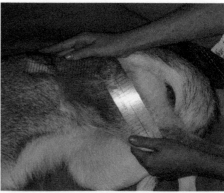

Fig. 3. A 1-year-old Siberian husky is evaluated for the left pelvic limb disuse after a femoral head ostectomy. The range of motion of the hip joint is evaluated using a plastic goniometer. Hip flexion (*left*) is 55° and hip extension (*right*) is 123°. Both flexion and extension are less than anticipated, reflecting periarticular fibrosis. (*Photograph courtesy of* D Marcellin-Little.)

evaluated, such as spins, glides, and distraction motions. These motions are small relative to flexion and extension, but nevertheless may provide valuable information in certain musculoskeletal conditions. Dogs sometimes circumduct, or wing in or out, during gait. Evaluation of these motions may also be useful.

Muscle Mass

Muscle atrophy and weakness are common after injury, and regaining muscle mass and strength are among the main goals of rehabilitation. Subjective evaluation of muscle atrophy is commonly performed by palpating both limbs simultaneously while the animal is in a standing position. Experienced evaluators can detect relatively subtle differences. More objective methods include dual-energy x-ray absorptiometry, magnetic resonance imaging, quantitative computerized tomography, and ultrasound (US) measurement of muscle mass. These methods are relatively expensive and may require heavy sedation or anesthesia. A practical method is to measure limb circumference using a spring-tension tape measure (**Fig. 4**). Measurements made without a spring-tension tape measure are inaccurate because the end tension of the tape depends on the subjective tensioning of the evaluator. A spring tension allows a consistent amount of end tension to be applied. In addition, specific bony landmarks must be used to establish the area of circumference measurement. Estimating the region of measurement or using soft tissue landmarks, such as the fold of the flank, result in inaccurate and inconsistent measurements and should not be used.

A muscle condition score has also been developed for cats that evaluates muscle mass, which can be independent of body fat content.[42] Evaluation of muscle mass includes visual examination and palpation over temporal bones, scapulae, lumbar vertebrae, and pelvic bones. A similar scoring system may be valid for dogs.

More objective methods of assessing muscle mass include measurement of limb circumference. Four devices were evaluated for measuring limb circumference at 4 locations on the canine hindlimb and forelimb.[43] Repeated measurements were made by multiple observers at the mid thigh, tibial tuberosity, the hock, and carpus bilaterally. Measurements with a spring tension tape measure and a retractable tape measure resulted in significantly smaller values at each site than an ergonomic measuring tape and a circumference measuring tape. Interobserver variation was

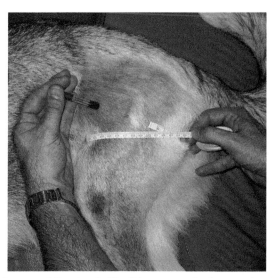

Fig. 4. The circumference of the dog in **Fig. 3** is measured using a spring-tension tape measure. The circumference was 31 cm on the left (affected side, pictured) and 35 cm on the opposite side. (*Photograph courtesy of* D Marcellin-Little.)

3.6 times greater than intraobserver variation. These results illustrate the importance of consistency when obtaining these measurements. The spring tension tape measure allows a constant end tension to be applied, eliminating subjective interpretation of how snug to pull the tape measure. In addition, specific anatomic landmarks and proper application of the tape measure can give repeatable readings between observers when using careful attention to detail.[44]

Measurement of muscle strength is more challenging. Although muscle mass and muscle strength are related, there is not a perfect correlation. Assessment of muscle strength in people is based on maximal effort to lift a load. This requires conscious knowledge of the task at hand. Because dogs cannot be instructed to provide maximum effort against a load, they must be coaxed or motivated to do so. This is difficult to do so consistently in an individual, no less in a group of dogs. Muscle maximal isometric extension torque has been measured in dogs, but requires anesthesia and placement of electrodes near motor nerves.[45]

Body Condition

Body condition, including lean tissue mass and body fat, has been measured with dual-energy x-ray absorptiometry, electrical impedance, and isotope dilution. These are impractical for clinical use, and body condition scoring performed by experienced evaluators has good correlation with more objective means.[46,47] However, owners often underestimate their dog's body condition score, making it important that an experienced person does the assessment.

Pain Assessment

Assessing pain is important in veterinary rehabilitation and methods of evaluation have been a focus of investigation. Although physiologic parameters have been investigated, these are most useful for assessing acute pain, such as immediately postoperatively. Evaluation of chronic pain has focused on behavioral characteristics. Ordinal and visual analog scores have been used to assess pain. Questionnaires have been developed that address specific areas of focus. The canine brief pain inventory is based on similar instruments used in people and has been validated in dogs with OA and bone cancer.[48–51] The Helsinki Chronic Pain Index was found to be a reliable tool to assess chronic pain by owners of dogs with OA.[52] Other pain assessment instruments are also available, including the Glasgow Composite Measure Pain Scale and the University of Melbourne Pain Scale, which evaluate features of acute pain.

Functional Scales

In addition to pain assessment, assessment of function has been evaluated, especially for spinal cord injury. A functional scoring system for dogs with acute spinal cord injuries is based on 5 stages of recovery of use of pelvic limbs. Each stage is subdivided based on recovery patterns, with a score of 0 to 14 possible.[53] The Texas Spinal Cord Injury Score for Dogs evaluates gait, proprioceptive positioning, and nociception. A score between 0 and 10 is possible.[54] A canine orthopedic index has also been developed and tested.[55–57] Additional validated scoring systems are needed in other areas, especially for orthopedic conditions other than OA.

THERAPEUTIC AND AQUATIC EXERCISES

Waining and others did a survey to determine the current status of canine hydrotherapy in the United Kingdom by sending a questionnaire to 152 hydrotherapy centers throughout the United Kingdom.[58] Although only 89 responded, they found that hydrotherapy was a rapidly growing business. Although stand-alone centers predominated, many hydrotherapy facilities were connected to other businesses, including boarding kennels and general veterinary practices. The most common conditions treated with hydrotherapy were ruptures of the cranial cruciate ligament (25%), hip dysplasia (24%), and OA (18%).

The complications from swimming in a chlorinated swimming pool were evaluated in 412 dogs.[59] The side effects included dry hair (20.63%), dry skin (18.93%), and abrasion wounds at the armpit (15.78%), all of which increased with greater frequency of swimming. Other adverse effects were red eye (13.59%), otitis (6.31%), and a small number of respiratory problems (0.49%).

The effect of water temperature on heart rate and respiratory rate during swimming was evaluated in 21 small breed dogs.[60] Dogs swam for 20 minutes in different water temperatures: 25, 33°C and 37°C. Heart rate and respiratory rate were monitored every 5 minutes during swimming. Blood samples were obtained before and after swimming for blood glucose and lactate concentrations. Dogs that swam in 25°C water had the highest heart rate and serum glucose levels. The highest respiration rate was found in dogs that swam in 37°C water. Serum lactate significantly increased after 20 minutes of swimming at all water temperatures. The authors suggested that dogs swim in 33°C water to prevent tachycardia, hyperventilation, and hyperthermia.

Changes in heart rate with swimming have been evaluated in small, medium, and large dogs.[61] Heart rates were measured every minute for 34 minutes after the fifth swimming session. Heart rates were significantly different between small, medium, and large dogs. An equation was developed that could predict heart rate of each group of dogs (small, medium, and large dogs). From their results, the authors recommended that the limits on the length of time swimming should be 15 to 30 minutes, depending on the breed (size) of dog.

Kinematic or motion analysis has been used to evaluate joint motion in dogs performing therapeutic exercises, including wheel-barrowing, dancing, incline and decline slope walking, ascending and descending stairs, Cavaletti walking, sit to stand, ground treadmill walking, underwater treadmill walking, and swimming.[62–65] Although there is a growing body of literature regarding normal dogs performing these exercises, additional information is needed regarding dogs with musculoskeletal issues performing these exercises and, more important, changes in response to rehabilitation.

THERAPEUTIC MODALITIES

Physical modalities are often used in the treatment of small animal patients. Modalities may be rather simple, suoh as cold and heat therapy, or more complex, such as NMES and extracorporeal shockwave therapy (ESWT). Therapeutic lasers are also increasingly used, and are the subject of an article by Pryor and Colleagues elsewhere in this issue. Although there is a relatively large volume of literature regarding the characteristics and use of modalities used in rehabilitation, there are relatively few studies in dogs, and most of these evaluate various characteristics of the modality, such as tissue temperature change with thermal modalities. There are even fewer studies evaluating clinical efficacy. Further, many clinicians combine several modalities in a single patient and there is virtually no information regarding whether combining modalities results in an additive, synergistic, or negative benefit.

Cryotherapy

Cryotherapy is often applied in the early postinjury or postoperative period to reduce blood flow, inflammation, swelling, and pain. Most studies of cryotherapy in dogs have focused on changes in tissue temperature. One study indicated that intra-articular temperature of the stifle joint of dogs decreased with increased time of cryotherapy application.[66] The greatest decrease in intra-articular temperature occurred in with ice water immersion. Rewarming of the stifle also took the longest with ice water immersion.

Cooling of different tissue depths for various times of cryotherapy application has also been investigated.[67] Skin and superficial tissues were cooled to the greatest extent. Deeper tissues had a more gradual decrease in tissue temperature. Rewarming was also slower in deeper tissues. Rewarming of tissues depends on the length of cryotherapy application. For example, muscle rewarming time to baseline temperatures was 60 minutes for 10 minutes of cryotherapy application time, 100 minutes for 15 minutes of application time, 130 minutes for 20 minutes of application time, 140 minutes for 25 minutes of application time, and 145 minutes for 30 minutes of application time. A study in our laboratory has shown similar results for cooling and rewarming at various tissue depths.[68] Millard and colleagues[69] also measured the effect of cold compress application on tissue temperature in 10 healthy, sedated dogs. Temperature changes were measured at 0.5, 1.0, and 1.5 cm tissue depths in a shaved, lumbar, epaxial region. Cold ($-16.8°C$) compresses were applied with gravity dependence for 5, 10, and 20 minutes. Temperature after 5 minutes of application at the superficial depth was significantly decreased, compared with control temperatures. Application for 10 and 20 minutes significantly reduced the temperature at all depths, compared with controls and 5 minutes of application. Twenty minutes of application significantly decreased temperature at only the middle depth, compared with 10 minutes of application. The authors concluded that 10 to 20 minutes of application caused a further significant temperature change at only the middle tissue depth; however, for maximal cooling, the minimum time of application should be 20 minutes. Changes in tissue temperature and adverse effects of application for longer than 20 minutes require further evaluation because it is possible that tissue damage may occur.

In a postoperative study of dogs undergoing extracapsular repair for cranial cruciate ligament rupture, cold compression and cold compression with bandaging were found to be equally beneficial in reducing stifle swelling in the first 72 hours.[70] Cold compression was applied for 20 minutes by wrapping the leg from the stifle to the hock with a large cold pack and holding it in place with an elastic bandage once daily.

Thermotherapy

There is relatively little information regarding heat therapy in dogs. In general, heat is used to increase blood flow, increase collagen extensibility, and perhaps provide some mild analgesia. In 1 study, the effect of warm compress application on tissue temperature in 10 healthy dogs was evaluated.[71] Tissue temperature was measured at depths of 0.5, 1.0, and 1.5 cm in a shaved lumbar, epaxial region in sedated dogs. Warm compresses (47°C) were applied with gravity dependence for 5, 10, and 20 minutes. After 5 minutes of heat application, tissue temperature at all depths was significantly increased, compared with the control temperatures. Application for 10 minutes resulted in even greater temperature at all depths, compared with 5 minutes of application. Tissue temperature with 20 minutes of application was not different at the superficial or middle depths, compared with 10 minutes of application. Overall, temperature increases at the deep depth were minimal. The authors suggested that application of a warm compress should be performed for 10 minutes. Changes in temperature at a tissue depth of 1.5 cm were minimal or not detected. However, the optimal compress temperature to achieve therapeutic benefits is still unknown.

Electrical Stimulation

Electrical stimulation has been used for many purposes in veterinary rehabilitation, including increasing muscle strength, muscle reeducation, increasing range of motion, pain control, accelerating wound healing, edema reduction, muscle spasm reduction, and enhancing transdermal administration of medication (iontophoresis). Transcutaneous electrical nerve stimulation (TENS) is widely recognized as a form of electrical stimulation that is used to modify pain, although technically nearly all clinical electrical stimulators elicit their actions through transcutaneous surface electrodes to stimulate nerves. Neuromuscular electrical nerve stimulation (NMES) or electrical muscle stimulation (EMS) is used for muscle reeducation, prevention of muscle atrophy, and to enhance joint movement.

For muscle strengthening, NMES creates a tetanic muscle contraction. NMES units have varying intensities and pulse durations to provide an electrical stimulus that results in depolarization of the motoneuron. A group of researchers determined the electrical impulse duration thresholds (chronaxy) for maximal motor contraction of various muscles without stimulation of pain fibers in dogs.[72] The chronaxy of a muscle is the pulse duration needed to obtain Aα fiber depolarization with an intensity value twice that of the rheobase (the intensity that causes Aα fiber depolarization when the pulse duration is $\geq$100 milliseconds). The chronaxy is important because it is the optimal pulse duration to cause depolarization of the Aα fibers and a resultant muscle contraction without recruiting nociceptive fibers. Eleven muscles were tested: Supraspinatus, infraspinatus, deltoideus, lateral head of the triceps brachii, extensor carpi radialis, gluteus medius, biceps femoris, semitendinosus, vastus lateralis, cranial tibial, and the erector spinae. The rheobase was used to determine the chronaxy for each of the 11 muscles in 10 dogs. Chronaxy values for stimulation of the biceps femoris, semitendinosus, and lower limb muscles were lower in dogs compared with humans. Chronaxy values did not differ between dogs and humans for the other muscles. Using specific chronaxy values for NMES should provide adequate stimulus for muscle strengthening with minimal stimulation of pain fibers.

The use of EMS has been studied in dogs recovering from surgical transection and subsequent stabilization of the cranial cruciate ligament-deficient stifle. In 1 study, dogs were subjected to an EMS treatment protocol for the thigh muscles 3 weeks after stabilization.[73] EMS-treated dogs had significantly better lameness score than did control dogs, with less palpable crepitation of the stifle, fewer degenerative radiographic changes, greater thigh circumference, and less gross cartilage damage. However, EMS-treated dogs had more medial meniscal damage, possibly as a result of increased limb use.

The effect of low-frequency NMES to increase muscle mass was studied in the quadriceps muscle of dogs with induced muscle atrophy.[74] Muscle atrophy was induced by immobilizing the left stifle joint for 30 days with transarticular external skeletal fixation. NMES began 48 hours after removal of the immobilization device, with dogs treated 5 times per week for 60 days at a frequency of 50 Hz, with pulse duration of 300 milliseconds, and an on/off time ratio of 1:2. Morphometry of vastus lateralis fibers obtained by muscle biopsy indicated a significant increase in muscle fiber transverse area of the treated group at 90 days compared with that identified at the time of immobilization. The authors concluded that low-frequency NMES results in hypertrophy of the vastus lateralis muscle in dogs after temporary rigid immobilization of the knee joint. Using the same model, these researchers also evaluated NMES at a frequency of 2500 Hz, with a pulse duration of 50%, and an on/off ratio of 1:2.[75] Although there was no difference between dogs receiving NMES and untreated controls regarding thigh circumference, cross-sectional morphometry of vastus lateralis fibers of treated dogs was greater on day 90 compared with that observed at the time of immobilization and untreated controls. Treated dogs also had improved goniometric measurements 30 days after immobilization ended. They concluded that this form of NMES also resulted in hypertrophy of the vastus lateralis muscle in dogs after induced muscular atrophy.

The effects of TENS have also been investigated in dogs with osteoarthritic pain in the stifle.[76] Five dogs with chronic mild OA were treated with premodulated electrical stimulation (70 Hz) applied to the affected stifle. Ground reaction forces were determined before treatment, immediately after treatment, and at 30-minute intervals over a 4-hour period. Significant improvement in ground reaction forces was found 30 minutes after treatment. These differences persisted for 210 minutes after TENS application and were significant 30, 60, 120, 150, and 180 minutes after treatment. However, the greatest improvement was found immediately after treatment. In this study, positive benefits of TENS application were apparent in dogs with osteoarthritic stifle joints.

The effects of low (TENS), medium (interferential), and high (microwave) electrotherapies on suppression of chronic pain in dogs with ankylosing spondylitis were studied.[77] Treatments were performed 15 minutes daily for 10 days. All groups had a significant decrease in pain at rest, during activity, or during palpation, with TENS having the greatest effect. Although all dogs improved clinically, none resulted in complete improvement of lameness.

Therapeutic Ultrasonography

Therapeutic ultrasound (US) is also commonly used in veterinary rehabilitation for its thermal and biologic effects. The thermal effects are especially beneficial for enhancing tissue extensibility, whereas the biologic effects may be useful for tissue and wound healing. Several studies have evaluated various properties of US treatment in dogs.

US energy does not transmit through air very well, and is best transmitted to the skin by clipping the hair to avoid trapped air and to use US coupling gel. US is also absorbed by tissues with high protein content, such as hair. A study was conducted in dogs to determine tissue temperature change when delivering US through intact, short, and clipped hair coats.[78] Heating of tissues did not occur with hair intact, despite using US gel on the hair and skin. The hair temperature increased, however. US delivered through short hair coats resulted in some tissue temperature increase, but the best results were obtained by clipping hair before US application.

One study examined tissue temperature changes of canine caudal thigh muscles at various depths during 3.3 MHz US treatments.[79] Dogs received 2 US treatments at intensities of 1.0 and 1.5 W/cm^2. Both intensities of US treatment were performed over a 10-cm^2 area for 10 minutes using a sound head with an effective radiating area of 5 cm^2. At the completion of the 10-minute US treatment the temperature rise at an intensity of 1.0 W/cm^2 was 3°C at the 1-cm depth, 2.3°C at 2 cm, and 1.6°C at 3.0 cm. At an intensity of 1.5 W/cm^2 tissue temperatures rose 4.6°C at the 1.0-cm depth, 3.6°C at 2 cm, and 2.4°C at 3 cm. Tissue temperature increases were gradual and cumulative over the time of US application. However, tissue temperatures returned to baseline within 10 minutes after treatment in all dogs, indicating that heating is relatively short lived.

The response of tendons to US treatment of tendons may differ from muscles because tendons are relatively smaller and have less blood supply. Four US treatments were randomly applied to the common calcaneal tendon of dogs: (1) Continuous US at 1.0 W/cm^2, (2) continuous US at 1.5 W/cm^2, (3) pulsed mode US at 1.0 W/cm^2, and (4) pulsed mode US at 1.5 W/cm^2.[80] Continuous mode US resulted in significantly greater tendon heating than pulsed US, and the magnitude of temperature increase should be safe for tissues. In addition, 1.5 W/cm^2 continuous US resulted in significantly greater tendon heating than 1 W/cm^2 continuous US. Mild increases in tendon temperature occurred with pulsed mode US (all <1.5°C), but there were no differences between 1 and 1.5 W/cm^2 pulsed mode US. The pattern of heating seems to be different between tendon and muscle. Although muscle has a relatively steady increase in tissue temperature during US treatment, tendon temperature in this study increased relatively rapidly within the first 2 minutes, and then stayed relatively constant for the remaining 8 minutes of treatment time. Increasing tendon extensibility with US was also studied. Using a standard amount of force, pre and post US treatment of the calcaneal tendon using 1.5 W/cm^2 continuous mode US resulted in significantly increased hock flexion immediately after treatment, but by 5 minutes after US, hock flexion returned to near baseline.

Extracorporeal Shockwave Therapy

Extracorporeal shockwaves are acoustic waves of high pressure and velocity that are delivered to tissues to produce biologic effects, including analgesia, neovascularization, production of growth factors, and improved tissue healing. There are 2 main types of ESWT units—focused and radial. Focused shockwave units have the ability to deliver the sound wave to a relatively small range of tissue depth, and units focus the energy to various depths using a variety of methods. The advantage of focused units is that the energy can be delivered to the area that requires treatment, and a relatively high amount of energy can be delivered. Radial shockwave units deliver the energy to the surface, and the energy waves spread out over a large volume of tissue. The sound energy is delivered to a relatively large amount of tissue, but if the target tissue is deep to the surface, much of the energy that is delivered dissipates by the time the sound reaches the intended region. Also, the therapist must be careful that there are truly sound waves that are being delivered because many of these devices merely deliver a mechanical concussive force. Clinically, ESWT has been used in people for the management of plantar fasciitis, lateral epicondylitis, calcifying tendinitis, femoral head necrosis, and the treatment of delayed union and nonunion fractures; in horses for insertion desmopathies, bone spavin, tendon and ligament calcification, navicular disease, exostoses, fractures and microfractures, back pain, and OA of tarsometatarsal and distal intertarsal joints; and in dogs for hypertrophic nonunions, tendonitis, spondylosis, and OA.

Mueller and coworkers[81] evaluated the effect of radial ESWT on dogs with hip OA. Dogs with hip OA were treated with EWST 3 times at weekly intervals. Six dogs with hip OA were not treated and served as controls. Ground reaction forces were obtained before and 6, 12, and 24 weeks after treatment. Treated dogs had a more symmetric gait; however, untreated dogs also had similar changes in peak vertical force at 6 weeks.

Results of analgesia were similar to a study of canine stifle OA, in which 3 shockwave treatments (200 shockwaves were applied to each of 4 sites using a 20-mm focused depth applicator, followed by 175 shocks to each of the same 4 sites using a 5-mm focused depth applicator, at an energy flux density of 0.14 mJ/mm, for a total of 1500 shocks) were administered 3 weeks apart.[82] Peak vertical force and vertical impulse were improved at 21 days and continued to improve to the end of the study, at 98 days. Despite these improvements, the changes were not significant from control groups, perhaps because of small numbers of animals in each group.

Our group reported significant improvement in ground reaction forces of dogs with elbow or hip OA compared with control groups.[83] A follow-up study of another group of dogs with elbow OA only confirmed these findings and suggested that the amount of improvement with ESWT is similar to what would be expected when treating with an average nonsteroidal anti-inflammatory drug (NSAID), although the dogs were already receiving treatment for their arthritis, including NSAIDs.[84]

ESWT also apparently has benefit in the treatment of tendon–bone and ligament–bone interface conditions. Evaluation of the bone–tendon interface in experimental dogs has revealed increased neovascularization after treatment, indicated by an increase in neovessels and angiogenic markers, such as vascular endothelial growth factor, endothelial nitric oxide synthase, and proliferating cell nuclear antigen expression.[85] ESWT was used for the treatment of supraspinatus calcifying tendinopathy in dogs. One dog had subjective and objective improvement in lameness 21 days after ESWT.[86] Another dog in the same report was bilaterally affected and improvement was noted 28 and 49 days after treatment in the right limb but not in the left limb. In both cases, disruption of the calcified material was not apparent after treatment. ESWT has also been evaluated for the treatment of patellar ligament desmitis in dogs after undergoing tibial plateau leveling osteotomy (TPLO).[87] Dogs that had TPLO surgery were evaluated preoperatively and 4, 6, and 8 weeks after TPLO. At 4 and 6 weeks, treated dogs received 600 shocks with an energy level of 0.15 mJ/mm^2 with a focused depth of application of 5 mm on the patellar ligament. There was a significant difference in distal patellar ligament thickness between groups at 6 and 8 weeks postoperatively.

One of the first uses for ESWT in people was the treatment of delayed and nonunion fractures. In a radial nonunion model performed in dogs, 80% of the dogs exhibited a bridging callus 6 weeks after shockwave treatment; by 9 weeks, there was narrowing of the fracture gap and an increase in the bridging callus, and finally complete bony union 12 weeks after treatment.[88] Persistent radiographic nonunion was present in 4 of 5 of the control dogs, however. Wang and colleagues[89] described the effects of ESWT in an acute fracture model on 16 tibiae of 8 laboratory dogs. In this study, radiographic callus formation was not better than control specimens until 12 weeks after treatment. Cortical bone at 12 weeks was histologically denser, thicker, and heavier than control callus, signifying the potential advantage of treating acute fractures. Therefore, it can be assumed that ESWT treatment improves the quality and mechanical qualities of bone during fracture repair. Shockwave therapy is associated with decreased incidence of disturbed fracture healing, and may be indicated for use in patients with multiple fractures, open fractures, animals with a concurrent systemic disease, or geriatric animals.[90]

Pulsed Electromagnetic Fields

Pulsed electromagnetic fields (PEMF) have been used in the treatment of OA with mixed results. A clinical study evaluated the effects of PEMF on OA in dogs compared with the NSAID firocoxib.[91] Twenty-five dogs were treated with PEMF once a day and 15 dogs were treated with firocoxib once daily for 20 days. Blinded clinical examination and owner's assessment before and after the therapy, as well as 4 and 12 months later, indicated that both groups had decreased clinical signs of OA. In the PEMF group, the effects were sustained for the 12-month study, whereas the control group tended to return to baseline values after the end of the 20-day treatment. Unfortunately, there was no control group in this study that used only subjective evaluation methods.

One randomized, controlled, blinded, clinical trial of dogs suggested that pulsed signal therapy was useful in treating 60 patients with OA.[92] Dogs in the treatment group received PST for 1 hour on 9 consecutive days. Outcome measures were performed on days 0, 11, and 42. The PST group performed significantly better than the control group as measured by the Canine Brief Pain Inventory Severity and Interference scores. Joint extension and peak vertical force were not significant after adjusting for multiple comparisons. The authors concluded that the PST group performed better than the control group according to owner assessment. There was a trend toward improvement in the PST group for objective force plate assessment of gait.

It is possible that PEMF may potentiate the response to morphine analgesia after abdominal surgery. A randomized, controlled, clinical trial evaluated PEMF therapy on postoperative pain in dogs undergoing ovariohysterectomy.[93] Although no clear benefit was seen in this study, the results suggested that PEMF may augment morphine analgesia after ovariohysterectomy in dogs.

One of the original tenets in the clinical use of PEMF stems from the fact that bone has streaming electrical fields when loaded. Therefore, it is logical to assess whether the external use of PEMF aids bone healing. The effect of PEMF on the healing of experimental lumbar spinal fusions was evaluated in dogs.[94] After surgery, 1 group was stimulated with a pulse burst-type signal PEMF for 30 minutes a day, another group was stimulated with the same PEMF for 60 minutes a day, and a third group received no active PEMF stimulation. No difference in the radiographic or histologic appearance of the fusion mass could be detected between the stimulated and control groups, suggesting that PEMF stimulation had no effect on the healing of posterior spinal fusions in this canine model. However, PEMF used in the late phase of bone healing in a tibia defect model stimulated bone healing in dogs that were stimulated 1 hour per day for 8 weeks.[95] Callus area increased earlier in the PEMF group, and maximum torque, torsional stiffness, new bone formation in the osteotomy gap, and mineral apposition rate were greater in the PEMF group.

If PEMF has value in bone healing, other wounds may also benefit from treatment. The effects of PEMF on the healing of open and sutured wounds was evaluated in dogs.[96] Open and sutured skin wounds were created over the trunk of dogs. The PEMF-treated dogs received treatment twice a day starting the day before surgery and for 21 days after surgery. PEMF treatment resulted in enhanced epithelialization of open wounds 10 and 15 days after surgery. PEMF treatment also shortened wound contraction time.

REHABILITATION OF ORTHOPEDIC CONDITIONS
Cranial Cruciate Ligament Rupture

Rehabilitation is commonly performed after surgery for orthopedic patients, or as a part of conservative treatment of some orthopedic conditions. Understandably, the most information pertains to postoperative rehabilitation of cranial cruciate ligament rupture. One of the first studies regarding postoperative rehabilitation of dogs after extracapsular repair of naturally occurring cranial cruciate ligament rupture found that dogs receiving rehabilitation had improved stifle extension and thigh circumference compared with dogs not undergoing a rehabilitation program.[97] A large study also evaluated the relationship between stifle joint motion and lameness after TPLO surgery for dogs with cranial cruciate ligament rupture.[98] They found that loss of extension or flexion $\geq 10°$ was responsible for worse clinical lameness scores. Also, OA in the cranial femorotibial joint was associated with loss of stifle joint extension. Loss of extension or flexion should be assessed in dogs with persistent clinical lameness after TPLO so that early intervention can occur. This study provides guidelines to define clinically relevant loss of extension or flexion of stifle joint after TPLO.

A study of Labrador retrievers undergoing extracapsular repair followed by postoperative rehabilitation found that dogs had improved weight bearing as measured with force platform compared with those not undergoing rehabilitation.[99] Another study evaluated the influence of immediate physical therapy on the functional recovery of hind limbs of dogs with experimental cranial cruciate ligament rupture and surgical extracapsular stabilization.[100] The authors found that dogs undergoing immediate physical rehabilitation had better functional gait recovery. In addition, the therapeutic modalities used in the immediate postoperative period did not cause instability of the operated knee.

Another study evaluated the use of carprofen, an NSAID, during rehabilitation after extracapsular stabilization for cranial cruciate ligament rupture.[101] The results suggested that although both carpofen-treated and untreated dogs undergoing rehabilitation improved over time, carprofen treatment did not result in greater weight bearing, thigh circumference, range of motion, or perceived exertion. A similar study by the same group of researchers found similar results for the NSAID deracoxib, suggesting that NSAIDS during the chronic phase of rehabilitation may not be necessary.[102]

Other surgical procedures for stifle stabilization also apparently benefit from physical rehabilitation. A study evaluated the effects of early intensive postoperative physical rehabilitation on limb function in dogs after TPLO for cranial cruciate ligament rupture.[103] Six weeks after TPLO, the physical rehabilitation group had significantly larger thigh circumference than a home exercise group. In addition, the affected limb had the same thigh circumference as the unaffected limb, whereas differences persisted in the home exercise group. Stifle maximum extension and flexion were significantly greater in the physical rehabilitation group, compared with the home exercise group after surgery. The authors concluded that a properly managed early physical rehabilitation program after TPLO may help to prevent muscle atrophy, build muscle mass and strength, and increase stifle joint flexion and extension.

Another study of dogs undergoing either a home or professional rehabilitation program after extracapsular repair for cranial cruciate ligament rupture found no differences in outcome.[104] However, only subjective gait analysis, stifle stability by drawer motion, and thigh circumference were evaluated.

Short-term (3, 5, and 7 weeks postoperatively) and long-term (6 and 24 months) functional and radiographic outcomes of cranial cruciate ligament injury in dogs treated with postoperative physical rehabilitation and either TPLO or extracapsular repair were determined in 65 dogs.[105] The rehabilitation program was the same in both groups. Radiographic OA scores significantly progressed 24 months after surgery in all dogs. Peak vertical force increased from preoperative to 24 months postoperatively in both groups, and there were no differences between groups. Therefore, there were apparently no differences in outcome measures used in this study comparing 2 different surgical techniques with the same rehabilitation protocol. Unfortunately, groups not receiving rehabilitation were not studied.

Although intracapsular repair of cranial cruciate ligament rupture is not commonly performed, a study evaluated the influence of physical rehabilitation on functional stifle recovery and joint stability.[106] Eight dogs were allocated into control and rehabilitation groups. Rehabilitation was initiated immediately postoperatively, including cryotherapy, passive range of motion, massage, stretching, NMES, hot packs, and underwater treadmill walking. Therapeutic exercises included walks on grass and hard floor, ball, ramp, cones, obstacles, platform, and mattress. Gait evaluation, thigh circumference, stifle goniometry, hind limb and stifle radiography, and joint stability (drawer test) were assessed preoperatively and 45 and 90 days postoperatively. The authors concluded that rehabilitation immediately after intracapsular surgical reconstruction for cranial cruciate ligament rupture produced a satisfactory functional recovery and did not worsen stifle instability. Others have also evaluated the role of postoperative rehabilitation in experimental dogs receiving intracapsular repair. Muzzi and coworkers[107,108] evaluated the effect of physiotherapy after arthroscopic repair of the cranial cruciate ligament using an intracapsular arthroscopic technique with fascia lata as an autogenous graft. Eight dogs were included in a postoperative physiotherapy group and the other 8 in a temporary immobilization group. The first phase of study concluded that physiotherapy has beneficial effects on early limb function during the rehabilitation period. In the second part of the study they found that postoperative physiotherapy decreases degenerative joint disease progression and stimulates the incorporation of the graft.

Conservative management of cranial cruciate ligament instability is performed in some situations when surgery is not possible. Comerford and colleagues did a survey of cranial cruciate ligament rupture management in small dogs (<15 kg).[109] Immediate surgical management was chosen by 15.5% of the respondents, and 63.4% of those performed extracapsular stabilization, 32.9% corrective osteotomies and 6.8% intraarticular stabilization. Conservative management included NSAIDs (91.1%), short leash walks (91.1%), weight loss (89.0%), hydrotherapy (53.6%), physiotherapy (41.9%), and cage rest (24.2%). Based on the survey, they concluded that conservative management was still widely used for treatment of cranial cruciate ligament rupture in dogs weighting less than 15 kg. A prospective, randomized clinical trial of larger, overweight dogs with cranial cruciate rupture had either TPLO or conservative treatment, consisting of physical therapy, weight loss, and NSAIDs.[110] Although both groups improved on average, the surgically treated group had better peak vertical force than the conservative group at the later assessments. Surgical treatment group dogs had a higher probability of a successful outcome (67.7%, 92.6%, and 75.0% for the 12-, 24-, and 52-week evaluations, respectively) versus nonsurgical treatment group dogs (47.1%, 33.3%, and 63.6% for 12-, 24-, and 52-week evaluations, respectively).

Mostafa and coworkers evaluated the morphometric characteristics of the pelvic limb musculature of Labrador retrievers with and without cranial cruciate ligament deficiency, using radiography (widths of quadriceps, hamstrings and gastrocnemius were expressed relative to tibial length) and dual energy x-ray absorptiometry evaluation of the lean content of the same muscle groups.[111] They concluded that atrophy may predominantly affect the quadriceps muscle in affected dogs, and dominance of the gastrocnemius muscle over restraints to the cranial tibial thrust may be associated with predisposition to cranial cruciate ligament deficiency in Labrador retrievers. If confirmed, this dynamic imbalance between muscle groups of the rear limbs could serve as a basis for screening programs and preventive rehabilitation.

Osteoarthritis

Dogs with OA may also benefit from physical rehabilitation as part of the overall treatment program. Owners of Labrador retrievers with OA and restricted joint motion were given instructions for a home stretching program. Owners performed 10 passive stretches with a hold of 10 seconds twice daily. After 21 days, goniometric measurements showed that the passive stretching had significantly increased the range of motion of the joints by 7% to 23%.[112] The effects of a weight reduction program combined with a basic or more complex physical rehabilitation program on lameness in overweight dogs with OA was evaluated.[113] Caloric restriction combined with intensive physical rehabilitation improved mobility and facilitated weight loss in overweight dogs. The authors concluded that dietary management and physical rehabilitation may improve the health status more efficiently than dietary management alone.

Aquatic therapy may be especially useful for patients with OA because of the buoyancy, resistance, and hydrostatic pressure properties of water.[114] One study evaluated whether swimming improves function of osteoarthritic hip joints in dogs.[115] Fifty-five dogs were randomized to 1 of 3 groups: OA with swimming, non-OA with swimming, and non-OA without swimming. All animals were allowed to swim for a total of 8 weeks (2 days per week, with 3 cycles of swimming for 20 minutes, with a 5-minute rest period between cycles). Clinical evaluation of the OA with swimming group found that lameness, joint mobility, weight bearing, pain on palpation, and overall score were significantly improved at week 8 compared with pretreatment. Although an OA nonswimming group hindered definitive conclusions, the authors felt that swimming 2 days per week for 8 weeks can improve the function of joints with OA.

Muscles may play a role in joint adaptation, limb loading, and joint degeneration. Conversely, joint degeneration affects the control of muscle forces and joint position awareness. The changes in muscle forces acting on joints with OA have been studied experimentally in cats.[116] Cats with transection of the cranial cruciate ligament have decreased stifle extensor and hock extensor muscle forces, and reduced ground reaction forces. There are also changes in the muscle firing patterns and the coordination of extensor and flexor muscle groups while ambulating. These findings were then applied to studies regarding loading of articular cartilage by controlled nerve stimulation of muscle groups to create muscle forces that load joints.[116] The authors found that loading cat stifles for 30 to 60 minutes results in upregulation of messenger RNA of specific metalloproteinases and some of their inhibitors. Progressing further with a muscle weakness model using botulinum toxin injections in rabbit stifle extensor muscles, the authors were able to measure a 60% to 80% decrease in muscle force, which was associated with changes in external ground reaction forces.[116] More important, the muscle weakness seemed to be associated with degeneration of cartilage in the absence of joint instability. Based on their results, the researchers concluded that muscle health and muscle rehabilitation are key components in the prevention of, and recovery from, joint injury and disease.

Other articles have suggested rehabilitation protocols for various musculoskeletal conditions based on clinical experience in dogs and people, but the efficacy of these protocols has not been adequately studied.

REHABILITATION OF NEUROLOGIC CONDITIONS

The effect of physical rehabilitation was studied in dogs with degenerative myelopathy to evaluate whether mean survival time was significantly affected.[117] Animals that received intensive physiotherapy had longer survival time (mean, 255 days) compared with that for animals with moderate (mean, 130 days) or no (mean, 55 days) physiotherapy. In addition, the authors found that affected dogs that received physiotherapy remained ambulatory longer than did animals that did not receive physical treatment.

There is a report of successful treatment of a dog with traumatic cervical myelopathy treated with surgery, positive pressure ventilation, and physical rehabilitation, and another of 3 dogs with paresis or paralysis owing to compression of the caudal cervical spinal cord that were successfully treated with physiatry.[118,119]

Exercises have been described, along with their effects on mobilization of the lumbar spinal nerves and dura mater.[120] The clinical effects of these exercises have not been evaluated, however.

CONTRAINDICATIONS TO INTENSIVE REHABILITATION

The science of canine physical rehabilitation should consider every aspect of treatment because it is possible that physical rehabilitation may have unwanted outcomes. The effect of physical rehabilitation on dystrophin-deficient dogs was studied.[121] Golden retriever muscular dystrophy is a dystrophin-deficient canine model genetically homologous to Duchenne muscular dystrophy in humans. Muscular fibrosis secondary to cycles of degeneration/regeneration of dystrophic muscle tissue and muscular weakness leads to biomechanical adaptation that impairs the quality of gait. Physical therapy in people is controversial and there is no consensus regarding the type and intensity of physical therapy. In this study of dogs, the effect of physical rehabilitation on gait biomechanics and deposition of muscle collagen types I and III in dystrophin-deficient dogs was studied. Two dystrophic dogs underwent a rehabilitation protocol of active walking exercise, 3 times per week, 40 minutes per day, for 12 weeks. Two dystrophic control dogs maintained their routine of activities of daily living. The rehabilitation protocol accelerated morphologic alterations in dystrophic muscle and resulted in slower velocity of gait. Control dogs that maintained their routine of activities of daily living had a better balance between movement and preservation of motor function.

REFERENCES

1. Millis DL. Responses of musculoskeletal tissues to disuse and remobilization. In: Millis DL, Levine, editors. Canine Rehabilitation and Physical Therapy. Elsevier; 2014.

2. Kiviranta I, Jurvelin J, Tammi M, et al. Weight bearing controls glycosamino-glycan concentration and articular cartilage thickness in the knee joints of young beagle dogs. Arthritis Rheum 1987;30:801–9.
3. Palmoski MJ, Bean JS. Cartilage atrophy induced by limb immobilization. In: Greenwald RA, Diamond HS, editors. CRC handbook of animal models for the rheumatic diseases. Boca Raton (FL): CRC Press; 1988. p. 83–7.
4. Palmoski M, Perricone E, Brandt KD. Development and reversal of a proteogly-can aggregation defect in normal canine knee cartilage after immobilization. Arthritis Rheum 1979;22:508–17.
5. Haapala J, Arokoski J, Pirttimaki J, et al. Incomplete restoration of immobilization induced softening of young beagle knee articular cartilage after 50-week remo-bilization. Int J Sports Med 2000;21:76–81.
6. Palmoski MJ, Brandt KD. Running inhibits the reversal of atrophic changes in canine knee cartilage after removal of a leg cast. Arthritis Rheum 1981;24: 1329–37.
7. Grynpas MD, Kasra M, Renlund R, et al. The effect of pamidronate in a new model of immobilization in the dog. Bone 1995;17:225S–32S.
8. Waters DJ, Caywood DD, Turner RT. Effect of tamoxifen citrate on canine immo-bilization (disuse) osteoporosis. Vet Surg 1991;20:392–6.
9. Waters DJ, Caywood DD, Trachte GJ, et al. Immobilization increases bone pros-taglandin E. Effect of acetylsalicylic acid on disuse osteoporosis studied in dogs. Acta Orthop Scand 1991;62:238–43.
10. Jee WS, Ma Y. Animal models of immobilization osteopenia. Morphologie 1999; 83:25–34.
11. Marotti G, Delrio N, Marotti F, et al. Quantitative analysis of the bone destroying activity of osteocytes and osteoclasts in experimental disuse osteoporosis. Ital J Orthop Traumatol 1979;5:225–40.
12. Kaneps AJ, Stover SM, Lane NE. Changes in canine cortical and cancellous bone mechanical properties following immobilization and remobilization with ex-ercise. Bone 1997;21:419–23.
13. Jaworski ZF, Uhthoff HK. Reversibility of nontraumatic disuse osteoporosis dur-ing its active phase. Bone 1986;7:431–9.
14. Booth FW, Gould EW. Effects of training and disuse on connective tissue. Exerc Sport Sci Rev 1975;3:83–112.
15. Lieber RL, Friden JO, Hargens AR, et al. Differential response of the dog quadriceps muscle to external skeletal fixation of the knee. Muscle Nerve 1988;11:193–201.
16. Appell HJ. Muscular atrophy following immobilization. A review. Sports Med 1990;10:42–58.
17. Lieber RL, McKee WT, Gershuni DH. Recovery of the dog quadriceps after 10 weeks of immobilization followed by 4 weeks of remobilization. J Orthop Res 1989;7:408–12.
18. Francis DA, Millis DL, Head LL. Bone and lean tissue changes following cranial cruciate ligament transection and stifle stabilization. J Am Anim Hosp Assoc 2006;42:127–35.
19. Innes JF, Barr AR. Clinical natural history of the postsurgical cruciate deficient canine stifle joint: year 1. J Small Anim Pract 1998;39:325–32.
20. de Souza SF, Padilha JG, Martins VM, et al. Clinical aspects and serum concen-tration creatine kinase and lactate dehydrogenase in dogs submitted to physio-therapy after induced muscle atrophy. Ciencia Rural 2011;41:1255–61.
21. Yasuda K, Hayashi K. Changes in biomechanical properties of tendons and lig-aments from joint disuse. Osteoarthr Cartil 1999;7:122–9.

22. Klein L, Player JS, Heiple KG, et al. Isotopic evidence for resorption of soft tissues and bone in immobilized dogs. J Bone Joint Surg Am 1982;64:225–30.

23. Laros GS, Tipton CM, Cooper RR. Influence of physical activity on ligament insertions in the knees of dogs. J Bone Joint Surg Am 1971;53:275–86.

24. Tipton CM, James SL, Mergner WA. Influence of exercise on the strength of medial collateral ligaments of dogs. Am J Physiol 1970;218:894–902.

25. Michel KE, Brown DC. Determination and application of cut points for accelerometer-based activity counts of activities with differing intensity in pet dogs. Am J Vet Res 2011;72:866–70.

26. Swimmer RA, Rozanski EA. Evaluation of the 6-minute walk test in pet dogs. J Vet Intern Med 2011;25:405–6.

27. Hicks DA, Millis DL, Arnold GA, et al. Comparison of weight bearing at a stance vs. trotting in dogs with rear limb lameness. Proc of the 32nd Veterinary Orthopedic Society, Snowmass, CO, March 2005. p. 12.

28. Hyytiainen HK, Molsa SH, Junnila JT, et al. Use of bathroom scales in measuring asymmetry of hindlimb static weight bearing in dogs with osteoarthritis. Vet Comp Orthop Traumatol 2012;25:390–6.

29. Budsberg SC, Verstraete MC, Brown J, et al. Vertical loading rates in clinically normal dogs at a trot. Am J Vet Res 1995;56:1275–80.

30. DeCamp CE. Kinetic and kinematic gait analysis and the assessment of lameness in the dog. Vet Clin North Am Small Anim Pract 1997;27(4):825–40.

31. Korvick DL, Pijanowski GJ, Schaeffer DJ. Three-dimensional kinematics of the intact and cranial cruciate ligament-deficient stifle of dogs. J Biomech 1994;27:77–87.

32. Bockstahler BA, Prickler B, Lewy E, et al. Hind limb kinematics during therapeutic exercises in dogs with osteoarthritis of the hip joints. Am J Vet Res 2012;73:1371–6.

33. Bockstahler B, Fixl I, Dal-Bianco B, et al. Kinematical motion analysis of the front legs of dogs suffering from osteoarthritis of the elbow joint during special physical therapy exercise regimes. Wien Tierarztl Monatsschr 2011;98:87–94.

34. Foss K, da Costa RC, Rajala-Shultz PJ, et al. Force plate gait analysis in Doberman pinschers with and without cervical spondylomyelopathy. J Vet Intern Med 2013;27:106–11.

35. Gordon-Evans WJ, Evans RB, Knap KE, et al. Characterization of spatiotemporal gait characteristics in clinically normal dogs and dogs with spinal cord disease. Am J Vet Res 2009;70:1444–9.

36. Marsolais GS, McLean S, Derrick T, et al. Kinematic analysis of the hind limb during swimming and walking in healthy dogs and dogs with surgically corrected cranial cruciate ligament rupture. J Am Vet Med Assoc 2003;222:739–43.

37. Ragetly CA, Griffon DJ, Mostafa AA, et al. Inverse dynamics analysis of the pelvic limb in Labrador retrievers with and without cranial cruciate ligament disease. Vet Surg 2010;39:1–10.

38. Headrick JF, Zhang S, Millard RP, et al. Use of an inverse dynamics method to compare the three-dimensional motion of the pelvic limb among clinically normal dogs and dogs with cranial cruciate ligament–deficient stifle joints following tibial plateau leveling osteotomy or lateral fabellar–tibial suture stabilization. Am J Vet Res 2014;75:554–64.

39. Nielsen C, Stover SM, Schulz KS, et al. Two-dimensional link-segment model of the forelimb of dogs at a walk. Am J Vet Res 2003;64:609–17.

40. Jaegger G, Marcellin-Little DJ, Levine D. Reliability of goniometry in Labrador Retrievers. Am J Vet Res 2002;63:979–86.

41. Jaeger GH, Marcellin-Little DJ, DePuy V, et al. Validity of goniometric joint measurements in cats. Am J Vet Res 2007;68:822–6.

42. Michel KE, Anderson W, Cupp C, et al. Validation of a subjective muscle mass scoring system for cats. J Anim Physiol Anim Nutr (Berl) 2009;93:806.
43. Baker SG, Roush JK, Unis MD, et al. Comparison of four commercial devices to measure limb circumference in dogs. Vet Comp Orthop Traumatol 2010;23: 406–10.
44. Millis DL, Scroggs L, Levine D. Variables Affecting Thigh Circumference Measurements in Dogs. Proceedings of The First International Symposium on Rehabilitation and Physical Therapy in Veterinary Medicine. Corvallis, OR, August 1999.
45. Lieber RL, Jacks TM, Mohler RL, et al. Growth hormone secretagogue increases muscle strength during remobilization after canine hindlimb immobilization. J Orthop Res 1997;15:519–27.
46. German AJ, Holden SL, Moxham GL, et al. A simple, reliable tool for owners to assess the body condition of their dog or cat. J Nutr 2006;136:2031S–3S.
47. Laflamme D. Development and validation of a body condition score system for dogs. Canine Practice 1997;22:10–5.
48. Brown DC, Boston RC, Coyne JC, et al. Development and psychometric testing of an instrument designed to measure chronic pain in dogs with osteoarthritis. Am J Vet Res 2007;68:631–7.
49. Brown DC, Boston RC, Coyne JC, et al. Ability of the Canine Brief Pain Inventory to detect response to treatment in dogs with osteoarthritis. J Amer Vet Med Assoc 2008;233:1278–83.
50. Brown DC. Power of treatment success definitions when the Canine Brief Pain Inventory is used to evaluate carprofen treatment for the control of pain and inflammation in dogs with osteoarthritis. Amer J Vet Res 2013;75:1467–73.
51. Brown DC, Boston R, Coyne JC, et al. A Novel Approach to the Use of Animals in Studies of Pain: Validation of the Canine Brief Pain Inventory in Canine Bone Cancer. Pain Med 2009;10:133–42.
52. Hielm-Björkman AK, Rita H, Tulamo R-M. Psychometric testing of the Helsinki chronic pain index by completion of a questionnaire in Finnish by owners of dogs with chronic signs of pain caused by osteoarthritis. Am J Vet Res 2009; 70:727–34.
53. Olby NJ, De Risio L, Muñana KR, et al. Functional scoring system in dogs with acute spinal cord injuries. Am J Vet Res 2001;62:1628.
54. Levine GJ, Levine JM, Budke CM, et al. Description and repeatability of a newly developed spinal cord injury scale for dogs. Prev Vet Med 2009;89:121–7.
55. Brown DC. The Canine Orthopedic Index. Step 1: devising the items. Vet Surg 2014;43:232–40.
56. Brown DC. The Canine Orthopedic Index. Step 2: psychometric testing. Vet Surg 2014;43:241–6.
57. Brown DC. The Canine Orthopedic Index. Step 3: responsiveness testing. Vet Surg 2014;43:247–54.
58. Waining M, Young IS, Williams SB. Evaluation of the status of canine hydrotherapy in the UK. Vet Rec 2011;168:407.
59. Nganvongpanit K, Yano T. Side effects in 412 dogs from swimming in a chlorinated swimming pool. Thai J Vet Med 2012;42:281–6.
60. Nganvongpanit K, Boonchai T, Taothong O, et al. Physiological effects of water temperatures in swimming toy breed dogs. Kafkas Univ Vet Fak Deg 2014;20: 177–83.
61. Nganvongpanit K, Kongsawasdi S, Chuatrakoon B, et al. Heart rate change during aquatic exercise in small, medium and large healthy dogs. Thai J Vet Med 2011;41:455–61.

62. Feeney LC, Lin CF, Marcellin-Little DJ, et al. Validation of two-dimensional kinematic analysis of walk and sit-to-stand motions in dogs. Am J Vet Res 2007;68: 277–82.

63. Holler PJ, Brazda V, Dal-Bianco B, et al. Kinematic motion analysis of the joints of the forelimbs and hind limbs of dogs during walking exercise regimens. Am J Vet Res 2010;71:734–40.

64. Hicks DA, Millis DL, Schwartz P, et al. Kinematic assessment of selected therapeutic exercises in dogs. 3rd International Symposium on Physical Therapy and Rehabilitation in Veterinary Medicine, Raleigh, NC, August, 2004.

65. Weigel JP, Millis DL. Biomechanics of physical rehabilitation and kinematics. In: Millis DL, Levine D, editors. Canine Rehabilitation and Physical Therapy. Elsevier; 2014.

66. Bocobo C, Fast A, Kingery W, et al. The effect of ice on intra-articular temperature in the knee of the dog. Am J Phys Med Rehabil 1991;70:181–5.

67. Akgun K, Korpinar MA, Kalkan MT, et al. Temperature changes in superficial and deep tissue layers with respect to time of cold gel pack application in dogs. Yonsei Med J 2004;45:711–8.

68. Vannatta ML, Millis DL, Adair S, et al. Effects of cryotherapy on temperature change in caudal thigh muscles of dogs. 31st Veterinary Orthopedic Society, Big Sky, MT, February 2004.

69. Millard RP, Towle-Millard HA, Rankin DC, et al. Effect of cold compress application on tissue temperature in healthy dogs. Am J Vet Res 2013;74:443–7.

70. Rexing J, Dunning D, Siegel AR, et al. Effects of cold compression, bandaging, and microcurrent electrical therapy after cranial cruciate ligament repair in dogs. Vet Surg 2010;39:54–8.

71. Millard RP, Towle-Millard HA, Rankin DC, et al. Effect of warm compress application on tissue temperature in healthy dogs. Am J Vet Res 2013;74:448–51.

72. Sawaya SG, Combet D, Chanoit G, et al. Assessment of impulse duration thresholds for electrical stimulation of muscles (chronaxy) in dogs. Am J Vet Res 2008;69:1305–9.

73. Johnson JM, Johnson AL, Pijanowski GJ. Rehabilitation of dogs with surgically treated cranial cruciate ligament deficient stifles by use of electrical stimulation of muscles. Am J Vet Res 1997;58:1473–8.

74. Pelizzari C, Mazzanti A, Raiser AG, et al. Neuromuscular electric stimulation in dogs with induced muscle atrophy. Arq Bras Med Vet Zootec 2008;60:76–82.

75. Pelizzari C, Mazzanti A, Raiser AG, et al. Medium frequency neuromuscular electrical stimulation (Russian) in dogs with induced muscle atrophy. Ciência Rural 2008;38:736–42.

76. Johnston KD, Levine D, Price MN, et al. The Effect of Tens on Osteoarthritic Pain in the Stifle of Dogs. Proc 2nd International Symposium on Physical Therapy and Rehabilitation in Veterinary Medicine, Knoxville, TN, August, 2002.

77. Krstic N, Lazarevic-Macanovic M, Prokic B, et al. Testing the effect of different electrotherapeutic procedures in the treatment of canine ankylosing spondylitis. Acta Vet Brno 2010;60:585–95.

78. Steiss JE, Adams CC. Rate of temperature increase in canine muscle during 1 MHz ultrasound therapy: deleterious effect of hair coat. Am J Vet Res 1999;60:76–80.

79. Levine D, Millis DL, Mynatt T. Effects of 3.3 MHz ultrasound on caudal thigh muscle temperature in dogs. Vet Surg 2001;30:170–4.

80. Loonam J, Millis DL, Stevens M, et al. The effect of therapeutic ultrasound on tendon heating and extensibility. In: Proceedings of the 30th Veterinary Orthopedic Society. Steamboat Springs (CO): 2003.

81. Mueller M, Bockstahler B, Skalicky M, et al. Effects of radial shockwave therapy on the limb function of dogs with hip osteoarthritis. Vet Rec 2007;160:762–5.

82. Dahlberg J, Fitch G, Evans RB, et al. The evaluation of extracorporeal shockwave therapy in naturally occurring osteoarthritis of the stifle joint in dogs. Vet Comp Orthop Traumatol 2005;18:147–52.

83. Francis DA, Millis DL, Evans M, et al. Clinical evaluation of extracorporeal shock wave therapy for management of canine osteoarthritis of the elbow and hip joint. In: Proceedings of the 31st Annual Conference Veterinary Orthopedic Society. Big Sky (MT): 2004.

84. Millis DL, Drum M, Whitlock D. Complementary use of extracorporeal shock wave therapy on elbow osteoarthritis in dogs. Vet Comp Orthop Traumatol 2011;24(3):A1.

85. Wang CJ, Huang HY, Pai HC. Shock wave-enhanced neovascularization at the tendon-bone junction an experiment in dogs. J Foot Ankle Surg 2001;14:17–21.

86. Danova NA, Muir P. Extracorporeal shock wave therapy for supraspinatus calcifying tendonopathy in two dogs. Vet Rec 2003;152:208–9.

87. Gallagher A, Cross AR, Sepulveda G. The effect of shock wave therapy on patellar ligament desmitis after tibial plateau leveling osteotomy. Vet Surg 2012;41:482–5.

88. Johannes EJ, Kaulesar Sukul DM, Matura E. High energy shock waves for the treatment of nonunions: an experiment in dogs. J Surg Res 1994;57:246–52.

89. Wang CJ, Huang HY, Chen HH, et al. Effect of shock wave therapy on acute fractures of the tibia. Clin Orthop Rel Res 2001;387:112–8.

90. Laverty PH, McClure SR. Initial experience with extracorporeal shock wave therapy in six dogs—part I. Vet Comp Orthop Traumatol 2002;15:177–83.

91. Pinna S, Landucci F, Tribuiani AM, et al. The effects of pulsed electromagnetic field in the treatment of osteoarthritis in dogs: clinical study. Pak Vet J 2013;33:96–100.

92. Sullivan MO, Gordon-Evans WJ, Knap KE, et al. Randomized, controlled clinical trial evaluating the efficacy of pulsed signal therapy in dogs with osteoarthritis. Vet Surg 2013;42:250–4.

93. Shafford HL, Hellyer PW, Crump KT, et al. Use of a pulsed electromagnetic field for treatment of post-operative pain in dogs: a pilot study. Vet Anaesth Analg 2002;29(1):43–8.

94. Khanaovitz N, Arnoczky SP, Nemzek J, et al. The effect of electromagnetic pulsing on posterior lumbar spinal fusions in dogs. Spine 1994;19:705–9.

95. Inoue N, Ohnishi I, Chen D, et al. Effect of pulsed electro- magnetic fields (PEMF) on late-phase osteotomy gap healing in a canine tibial model. J Orthop Res 2002;20:1106–14.

96. Scardino MS, Swaim SF, Sartin EA, et al. Evaluation of treatment with a pulsed electromagnetic field on wound healing, clinicopathologic variables, and central nervous system activity of dogs. Am J Vet Res 1998;59:1177–81.

97. Millis DL, Levine D, Weigel JP. A preliminary study of early physical therapy following surgery for cranial cruciate ligament rupture in dogs. Vet Surg 1997;26:254.

98. Jandi AS, Schulman AJ. Incidence of motion loss of the stifle joint in dogs with naturally occurring cranial cruciate ligament rupture surgically treated with tibial plateau leveling osteotomy: longitudinal case study of 412 cases. Vet Surg 2007;36:114–21.

99. Marsolais GS, Dvorak G, Conzemius MG. Effects of postoperative rehabilitation on limb function after cranial cruciate ligament repair in dogs. J Am Vet Med Assoc 2002;220:1325–30.

100. Berte L, Mazzanti A, Salbego FZ, et al. Immediate physical therapy in dogs with rupture of the cranial cruciate ligament submitted to extracapsular surgical stabilization. Arquivo Brasilerio de Medicina Veterinaria e Zootecnia 2012;64:1–8.
101. Gordon-Evans WJ, Dunning D, Johnson AL, et al. Effect of the use of carprofen in dogs undergoing intense rehabilitation after lateral fabellar suture stabilization. J Am Vet Med Assoc 2011;239:75–80.
102. Gordon-Evans WJ, Dunning D, Johnson AL, et al. Randomised controlled clinical trial for the use of deracoxib during intense rehabilitation exercises after tibial plateau leveling osteotomy. Vet Comp Orthop Traumatol 2010;23:332–5.
103. Monk ML, Preston CA, McGowan CM. Effects of early intensive postoperative physiotherapy on limb function after tibial plateau leveling osteotomy in dogs with deficiency of the cranial cruciate ligament. Am J Vet Res 2006;67:529–36.
104. Jerre S. Rehabilitation after extra-articular stabilization of cranial cruciate ligament rupture in dogs. Vet Comp Orthop Traumatol 2009;22:148–52.
105. Au KK, Gordon-Evans WJ, Johnson AL, et al. Comparison of short and long term function and radiographic osteoarthrosis in dogs receiving postoperative physical rehabilitation and tibial plateau leveling osteotomy or lateral fabellar suture stabilization. Vet Surg 2010;39:173–80.
106. Berte L, Salbego FZ, Baumhardt R, et al. Physiotherapy after cranial cruciate ligament replacement in dogs by using a homologous bone tendon segment preserved in 98% glycerin. Acta Scientiae Veterinariae 2014;42:1194.
107. Muzzi LA, Rezende CMF, Muzzi RAL. Physiotherapy after arthroscopic repair of the cranial cruciate ligament in dogs. I - clinical, radiographic, and ultrasonographic evaluation. Arq Bras Med Vet Zootec 2009;61:805–14.
108. Muzzi LA, Rezende CM, Muzzi RA. Physiotherapy after arthroscopic repair of the cranial cruciate ligament in dogs. II - Arthroscopic and anatomopathological evaluations. Arq Bras Med Vet Zootec 2009;61:815–24.
109. Comerford E, Forster K, Gorton K, et al. Management of cranial cruciate ligament rupture in small dogs: A questionnaire study. Vet Comp Orthop Trauma 2013;26:493–7.
110. Wucherer KL, Conzemius MG, Evans R, et al. Short-term and long-term outcomes for overweight dogs with cranial cruciate ligament rupture treated surgically or nonsurgically. J Am Vet Med Assoc 2013;242:1364–72.
111. Mostafa AA, Griffon DJ, Thomas MW, et al. Morphometric Characteristics of the Pelvic Limb Musculature of Labrador Retrievers with and without Cranial Cruciate Ligament Deficiency. Vet Surg 2010;39:380–9.
112. Crook T, McGowan C, Pead M. Effect of passive stretching on the range of motion of osteoarthritic joints in 10 Labrador retrievers. Vet Rec 2007;160:545–7.
113. Mlacnik E, Bockstahler BA, Müller M, et al. Effects of caloric restriction and a moderate or intense physiotherapy program for treatment of lameness in overweight dogs with osteoarthritis. J Am Vet Med Assoc 2006;229:1756–60.
114. Levine D, Marcellin-Little DJ, Millis DL, et al. Effects of partial immersion on vertical ground reaction forces and weight distribution in dogs. Am J Vet Res 2010;71:1413–6.
115. Nganvongpanit K, Tanvisut S, Yano T, et al. Effect of swimming on clinical functional parameters and serum biomarkers in healthy and osteoarthritic dogs. ISRN Vet Sci 2014;2014:459809. http://dx.doi.org/10.1155/2014/459809 eCollection.
116. Herzog W, Longino D, Clark A. The role of muscles in joint adaptation and degeneration. Langenbecks Arch Surg 2003;288:305–15.

117. Kathmann I, Cizinauskas S, Doherr MG, et al. Daily controlled physiotherapy increases survival time in dogs with suspected degenerative myelopathy. J Vet Intern Med 2006;20:927–32.
118. Smarick SD, Rylander H, Burkitt JM, et al. Treatment of traumatic cervical myelopathy with surgery, prolonged positive-pressure ventilation, and physical therapy in a dog. J Am Vet Med Assoc 2007;230:370–4.
119. Speciale J, Fingeroth JM. Use of physiatry as the sole treatment for three paretic or paralyzed dogs with chronic compressive conditions of the caudal portion of the cervical spinal cord. J Am Vet Med Assoc 2000;217:43–7, 29.
120. Gruencnfoldor FI, Boos A, Mouwen M, et al. Evaluation of the anatomic effect of physical therapy exercises for mobilization of lumbar spinal nerves and the dura mater in dogs. Am J Vet Res 2006;67:1773–9.
121. Gaiad TP, Araujo KPC, Serrao JC, et al. Motor physical therapy affects muscle collagen type I and decreases gait speed in dystrophin-deficient dogs. PLoS One 2014;9(4):e93500.

Physical Agent Modalities in Physical Therapy and Rehabilitation of Small Animals

June Hanks, PT, PhD, DPT, CWS, CLT[a],
David Levine, PT, PhD, DPT, CCRP, Cert. DN[a,*],
Barbara Bockstahler, Dr Vet Med, DVM, PD, CCRP[b]

KEYWORDS

- Superficial heat • Cryotherapy • Ultrasound • Physical agent modalities
- Electrotherapeutic modalities • Electrical stimulation • Cold packs • Hot packs

KEY POINTS

- Physical agent modalities are a useful adjunct to medical and surgical interventions, exercise, and manual therapy in the rehabilitation of animals.
- The most appropriate modality depends on the diagnosis, stage of healing, and treatment goals.
- Cold therapy is indicated in the management of acute injury or inflammation and for pain.
- Superficial heating agents such as hot packs penetrate to a tissue depth of approximately 2 cm, whereas deep heating with ultrasound can penetrate up to 5 cm.
- Heating agents are useful to increase tissue pliability and to decrease pain and muscle spasm.

INTRODUCTION

Physical agent modalities (PAMs) have been used in rehabilitation and physical therapy for centuries to reduce swelling, relieve pain, enhance healing, increase muscle strength, improve muscle tone, and affect the elasticity of connective tissue. Often used as a complement to therapeutic exercise in addition to medical and surgical interventions, PAMs assist to limit impairments and disability and to maximize function. The mechanism of action and depth of penetration varies with the method of application and the form of energy used. For example, direct contact between objects of

---

[a] Department of Physical Therapy, University of Tennessee at Chattanooga, 615 McCallie Avenue, Department #3253, Chattanooga, TN 37403, USA; [b] Section for Physical Therapy and Rehabilitation, Small Animal Surgery, Department for Small Animals and Horses, University of Veterinary Medicine Vienna, Wien A-1210, Austria
* Corresponding author.
E-mail address: David-Levine@utc.edu

Vet Clin Small Anim 45 (2015) 29–44
http://dx.doi.org/10.1016/j.cvsm.2014.09.002
0195-5616/15/$ – see front matter © 2015 Elsevier Inc. All rights reserved.
vetsmall.theclinics.com

different temperature can lead to thermal energy transfer through direct interaction of the molecules (conduction, as with hot/cold pack), through movement of fluid or air molecules across tissue interfaces (convection, as with hot or cold whirlpool), or through the transformation of nonthermal forms of energy such as sound waves to heat (conversion, as with ultrasound [US]).[1,2] Electrical stimulation (ES) is used primarily to treat acute and chronic pain and muscle atrophy. The purpose of this article is to review the use of cold, superficial heat, therapeutic US, and ES in small animal rehabilitation.

COLD (CRYOTHERAPY)
Basic Properties

Cryotherapy is the therapeutic application of cold in rehabilitation and physical therapy. Cold can be applied through a variety of mechanisms including cold packs, ice massage, cold water baths, mechanical and electrical compression units, and vapocoolant sprays. Cryotherapy can be used throughout the rehabilitative process to mitigate negative effects of inflammatory responses. Physiologically, local application of cold causes many changes, including temporary decreases in[3]:

- blood flow to the area
- edema formation
- hemorrhage
- histamine release
- local metabolism
- muscle spindle activity
- nerve conduction velocity (NCV)
- pain

In response to cooling, acutely inflamed tissues exhibit a slowed metabolic rate, inhibition of inflammatory enzymatic reactions, and reduced release of histamine. These physiologic responses serve to limit tissue damage.[4] The vasoconstriction associated with cold application limits edema formation and hemorrhage.[4–6] Pain may be lessened by reduced pressure on nociceptive receptors through edema reduction, and through reduced NCV.[7] In general, cold compresses should be applied for 10 to 20 minutes for therapeutic benefit.[8]

Indications

Cold is typically indicated in small animal rehabilitation for the management of acute injury or inflammation. PRICE is an acronym commonly used for acute injuries, and stands for Protection, Rest (to halt further injury), Ice (to decrease tissue metabolism and minimize tissue damage), Compression (to decrease edema), and Elevation (to decrease edema). In animals with acute injury, rest and ice can be readily used. Compression bandages may be applied to certain sites, such as a limb or distal joint such as the elbow, carpus, or stifle. Elevation is possible by keeping the edematous side up when in lateral recumbency. Application of cold to minimize postsurgical swelling is also recommended.[9]

The reduction in pain and inflammation with cryotherapy may lead to increased range of motion (ROM) in affected joints.[10,11] Local cold application may reduce spasticity in spinal cord disorders.[12] Cooling may inhibit the extension of tissue damage with thermal burns, with greatest benefit occurring when a coolant is applied immediately after burn injury.[13] For treatment of burn injury, the temperature of the coolant should be considered. In a study of induced dermal burns in pigs, cool water (temperature of 12°–18°C) was of greater benefit than cold water (temperature 1°–8°C) in limiting tissue damage.[14]

Several studies have examined the effectiveness of cold application following surgery. One study demonstrated superior edema reduction with cold application with and without bandaging compared with bandaging alone during the 72 hours following surgical repair of the cranial cruciate ligament.[9] Another study demonstrated reduced pain and swelling and increased motion in the stifle joint with cold application following tibial plateau-leveling osteotomy in dogs.[11]

Contraindications and Precautions

There are relatively few contraindications (never use it) and precautions (use it with caution) for cryotherapy. The primary precaution is avoidance of frostbite. It is difficult to check skin color on dogs because of pigmentation and hair coat. To be safe and avoid prolonged application, inspect the skin every few minutes. Cryotherapy is rarely applied directly onto the animal, owing to possible discomfort and/or tissue damage. The use of a towel between the cold pack or ice pack and the skin is recommended. The towel may be either dry or moist; if moist, it will cool to a greater extent as liquid is a better thermal conductor than air. More research is needed in dogs to document the amount and duration of tissue cooling with various forms of cold application. The insulating effect of the hair coat in dogs may be a factor to consider, although one study indicated that the extent of caudal thigh muscle cooling was similar with clipped and unclipped hair coat when cold packs (2 parts ice, 1 part isopropyl alcohol) were applied.[15] Other precautions and contraindications include the presence of cardiac or respiratory disease, uncovered open wounds, and ischemic areas.

General Guidelines for Application of Cold

During cold application, the treated tissue should be observed periodically to assure that the tissue is not being damaged. Color changes in the skin include redness (normal response) and blanching or whitening (sign of vasoconstriction and potential tissue damage). The recommended method of cold application depends on the therapeutic goal, stage of healing, location and size of the area to be treated, and practicality.

Cold packs/ice packs

Many types of cold packs are commercially available (**Fig. 1**). Ice packs can be made placing crushed ice in a moist towel or in a plastic bag wrapped in a moist towel. An ice pack that conforms easily around irregularly shaped body parts such as a limb can be made by placing a mixture of 3 parts water to 1 part rubbing alcohol in a plastic bag and then in the freezer. Although the cooling effect is significantly greater with a 20-minute application of a cold pack, a therapeutic amount of cooling may occur within 10 minutes.[8]

The effect of cold compresses (−16°C [3°F]) was studied on epaxial muscles in dogs.[8] The compresses were applied for 5, 10, and 20 minutes in random fashion, and temperature changes at 0.5, 1.0, and 1.5 cm of tissue depth were measured. At 10 minutes, the cold decreased tissue temperature at 0.5-, 1.0-, and 1.5-cm depths 7°C, 4.7°C, and 4°C, respectively. At 20 minutes the cold further decreased tissue temperature to 8.2°C, 6.5°C, and 4.7°C at the respective depths. The differences between the 10-minute and 20-minute applications were significant, with the 20-minute treatment being greater, but applications of 10 minutes were sufficient for therapeutic cooling. Dogs used in this study were of ideal body condition, making the results a good guide, but not applicable to overweight or underweight dogs.[8]

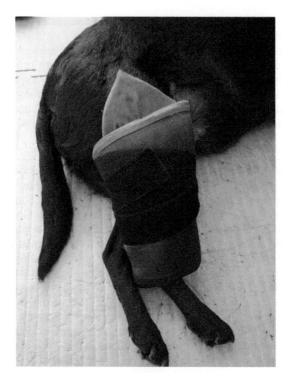

Fig. 1. Commercially available cold pack applied to the leg.

Cold-compression units
These commercially available devices consist of a sleeve with tubing running throughout that alternately circulates cold water and air. The combination of compression and cooling is effective in treating tissues in the acute phase of healing.

Cold immersion
In this type of application, the patient typically stands with the affected limb immersed in a container of cold water ($2°–16°C$). Rapid and significant tissue cooling occurs, but is difficult to apply because of poor patient compliance.

Ice massage
Water can be frozen in a Styrofoam or plastic cup and then applied to the affected area directly. To perform the massage, the therapist exposes a portion of the ice surface, holds the cup, and applies the ice surface directly to the patient's skin (**Fig. 2**). The ice surface is moved in a continuous, circular fashion across the treatment area for 5 to 10 minutes.

Cold application over casts or bandages
Superficial skin temperatures can be reduced with cold application over a cast or bandages. A greater decrease in skin temperature is observed with cold application over plaster and synthetic casts than over a bulky Robert-Jones dressing.[16,17]

HEAT

Heating agents are classified as superficial or deep heating. Superficial heating agents penetrate up to approximately 2 cm tissue depth, whereas deep heating agents

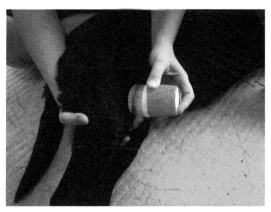

Fig. 2. During ice massage, the ice surface should be moved across the skin surface in a continuous, circular motion for 5 to 10 minutes.

elevate tissue temperatures at depths of 3 cm or more (**Table 1**). Heat sources are classified as radiant, conductive, or convective. An infrared lamp is an example of a radiant, superficial heating device. A hot pack is an example of a conductive, superficial heating device, and a whirlpool is an example of moist heat delivered by conduction and convection.

Basic Properties and Treatment Variables

Both heat and cold may be used for pain relief and reduction in muscle spasm, although the mechanism of action differs. Heat application causes increased:

- Vasodilation
- Tissue elasticity
- Muscle relaxation
- Pain relief

Locally applied superficial heating agents such as hot packs, electrical heating pads, and infrared lamps stimulate vasodilation through activation of bradykinin and nitrous oxide in the smooth muscle of blood vessels and through a reactive inhibition of sympathetic output. NCV increases, resulting in a decrease in pain and muscle spasm.[18]

Locally heated tissue increases in extensibility, thus reducing joint stiffness and leading to increased ROM. When soft tissue is heated before stretching, gains in tissue length are greater per unit force in achieving the length gain, and are maintained for longer periods of time than without prior heating.[18,19]

Therapeutic US has been used in small animal practice for a variety of purposes. Though primarily thought of as a deep heating agent,[20,21] it is also used for tissue

Table 1 Superficial versus deep heating agents	
Physical Agent	**Depth of Penetration**
Hot packs	Skin and down to 1.5 cm
Therapeutic ultrasound (3.3 MHz)	1.0–3.0 cm
Therapeutic ultrasound (1.0 MHz)	2.0–5.0 cm

healing and repair[22] and to enhance the transdermal administration of drugs (phonophoresis). The efficacy of phonophoresis has been reported in rats,[23–25] but studies in dogs are warranted.

US refers to high-frequency acoustic waves above the human hearing range (approximately 20 kHz). Sound waves are produced within a transducer head (also termed the sound head). The advantages of US are that it produces localized heating in deeper tissues and the duration of therapy is short, approximately 10 minutes. A disadvantage is that the heat is difficult to monitor exactly.

Indications

US is primarily used for the therapeutic effect of tissue temperature increase that leads to increased blood flow, decreasing pain and muscle spasm, improving collagen extensibility, and increasing ROM.

Contraindications and Precautions

There are certain conditions under which US should not be utilized or should be used with caution:

- Directly over the heart or in animals with pacemakers
- Over areas where thrombophlebitis is present (or any risk of embolus)
- Over infected areas or neoplasms
- Over areas with decreased or absent sensation
- Over the carotid sinus
- Over a pregnant uterus
- Plastic and metal implants
- Over the epiphyseal area of growing bones
- Over the spinal cord after laminectomy

Frequency

The typical therapeutic US unit has 2 frequencies, 1.0 and 3.3 MHz. The frequency is chosen based on the depth of tissue the clinician is trying to affect. The 1.0-MHz unit penetrates to a depth of 2.0 to 5.0 cm and the 3.3-MHz unit penetrates to 1.0 to 3.0 cm (see **Table 1**). Knowledge of the anatomy of the tissues that are being treated, in addition to the depth of the particular aspect of the tissues, is important in choosing the frequency.

Intensity

Intensity on most US devices can range from 0 to 2.5 W/cm^2. In general, the higher the intensity, the greater the temperature increases (**Table 2**).[20] Intensities required to increase tissue temperature 2.0°C or more generally vary from 1.0 to 2.0 W/cm^2

Table 2		
Tissue temperature change in dog caudal thigh muscles with ultrasound after 10 minutes of treatment		
	1 W/cm^2	1.5 W/cm^2
Tissue temperature at 1 cm depth (°C)	3	4.6
Tissue temperature at 2 cm depth (°C)	2.3	3.6
Tissue temperature at 3 cm depth (°C)	1.6	2.4

Data from Levine D, Millis DL, Mynatt T. Effects of 3.3-MHz ultrasound on caudal thigh muscle temperature in dogs. Vet Surg 2001;30(2):170–4.

continuous-mode US for 5 to 10 minutes. To heat an area with substantial soft tissue, intensities as high as 2.0 W/cm^2 may be used. If there is less soft tissue, or if bone is close to the skin surface, lower intensities are appropriate. After selection of an initial intensity, the patient's tolerance to the heat produced by the US is the final determinant of intensity, although this may be difficult to determine in pets. Most dogs lie quietly during US treatment. However, dogs sometimes begin to move or otherwise seem uncomfortable after commencing US. Although it may appear that the dog just wants to change position and move around, any clear signs of distress such as whining and crying may indicate pain, and the intensity of the US should be reduced or the session interrupted or discontinued. The skin also should never turn red or be hot to the touch.

The hair coat in dogs treated with US presents a problem not encountered with human patients. The hair coat should be clipped and cleaned before treatment. One study examined the effects of hair coat in dogs.[21] Ultrasound delivered through short-hair or long-hair coats produced nontherapeutic, minimal temperature increases in the underlying tissues when compared with US after the hair had been clipped. In addition, there was considerable warming within the hair coat at the skin interface that could cause skin burns.

Mode

The mode of US (often called the duty cycle) is typically used at either 100% (continuous) or 20% (pulsed). Other modes are available on some devices, but have not been well researched. The 100% continuous mode is used for heating effect and to increase tissue extensibility. The 20% pulsed mode is used for promotion and acceleration of tissue healing.[26]

Treatment Time

Treatment time is based on 2 factors: the size of the area to be treated and the size of the US transducer head. For each transducer head that fits in the area to be treated, approximately 4 minutes of US should be delivered. After determining the precise area to be treated, the number of transducer heads needed to cover the area must be determined. For example, if one is performing US on epaxial muscles and 3 sounds heads completely cover the area, the treatment time is approximately 12 minutes. Transducer heads come in a variety of sizes from 1 to 10 cm^2. A larger transducer head is much more effective from a time perspective than a small transducer head if large areas are to be treated. When applying US, the sound head should be moved continuously in circular or longitudinal patterns at an approximate speed of 4.0 cm/second.

Coupling Agents

A coupling medium, such as commercially available water-soluble gels or a coupling gel pad cushion, must be placed between the sound head and the tissue surface. The US sound beam is transmitted through the coupling medium to the skin. When using a water-soluble gel, the gel is applied to the area to be treated and the sound head is placed in direct contact with the gel. When using a coupling gel pad (**Fig. 3**), the gel pad is placed over the area to be treated and the sound head is placed in direct contact with the gel pad. This direct coupling method is preferred over other methods such as immersion under water. In the water-immersion method, the part to be treated must be immersed in water, all air bubbles must be removed from the water, and the sound head must be maintained at a distance of 0.5 to 3.0 cm from the skin surface during treatment. Studies indicate less of an increase in tissue temperature with the water-immersion method in comparison with direct application of the sound head.[27,28]

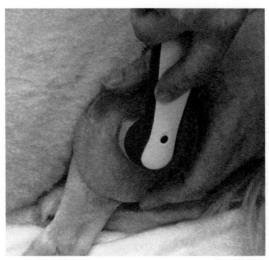

Fig. 3. A coupling gel pad is placed between the ultrasound head and the tissue to be treated.

Research on Ultrasound and Tissue Heating

One prospective randomized trial examined tissue temperature changes that occur at various depths during 3.3-MHz US treatments of the caudal thigh muscles in dogs.[20] Dogs received 2 randomly selected US treatments at intensities of 1.0 and 1.5 W/cm². Thermistors were inserted in the muscles at depths of 1.0, 2.0, and 3.0 cm, directly under the US treatment area. Both intensities of US treatment were performed on each dog over a 10-cm² area for 10 minutes using a sound head with an effective radiating area of 5 cm². Tissue temperature was measured before, during, and after US treatment until tissue temperature returned to baseline. At the completion of the 10-minute US treatment, the temperature increase at an intensity of 1.0 W/cm² was 3°C at the 1-cm depth, 2.3°C at 2.0 cm, and 1.6°C at 3.0 cm. At an intensity of 1.5 W/cm², tissue temperatures rose 4.6°C at the 1.0-cm depth, 3.6°C at 2.0 cm, and 2.4°C at 3.0 cm. Tissue temperatures returned to baseline within 10 minutes after treatment in all dogs. This study demonstrated that significant heating occurs in muscle during 3.3-MHz US, but the effect is relatively short-lived.[20] Another in vivo trial on dogs found heating with 1.0-MHz US at a depth of 5.0 cm with intensities of 1.5 W/cm² (2.0°C increase) and 2.0 W/cm² (3.5°C increase).[21] This same study found no heating at 10.0 cm of depth in any condition, which is consistent with in vivo studies on humans. A depth of 5.0 cm is thought to be the relative maximum depth at which US can have therapeutic benefit.

Research on Ultrasound and Tissue Healing

Most studies performed on US for tissue healing have been on animal models and have involved creating experimentally induced wounds. The animals typically have normal circulation, a condition that should be considered when interpreting effectiveness of treatment. One study using dogs[22] reported that pulsed US at 0.5 W/cm² enhanced healing of the common calcanean tendon. The US treatment was started the third day after surgically severing the tendon, and was performed daily for 10 days. A comprehensive review of the use of US for soft-tissue repair, wound healing, and fracture healing has recently been published, but is beyond the scope of this article.[26]

ELECTRICAL STIMULATION
Basic Concepts of Electrical Stimulation

Electrical stimulation (ES) has many documented benefits in humans, including increasing muscle strength, increasing ROM, decreasing acute and chronic pain, reducing muscle spasm, and promotion of soft-tissue and fracture healing.[29] The study of ES in dogs has focused on pain control and muscle strengthening.

Contraindications and Precautions

There are certain conditions under which ES should not be utilized, or should be used with caution:

- High-intensity stimulation directly over the heart or ES in animals with pacemakers
- Animals with seizure disorders (use around the head and neck)
- In areas with impaired sensation
- Over areas of thrombosis or thrombophlebitis
- Over infected areas or neoplasms
- Any time that active motion is contraindicated
- Over the trunk of pregnant females

Preparation and Electrode Placement

To ensure good contact of the electrodes with the skin surface, the animals' hair should be carefully clipped. Most electrodes are self-adherent and stick to the skin. If rubber electrodes are used, a gel medium or water-soaked sponges can be used at the electrode-skin interface. Wetting of the skin with water or alcohol is required if brush-like needle pads are used (**Fig. 4**). The animal should be placed in a comfortable position before the start of treatment. Initial treatments should be of short duration and low intensity to allow the animal to become accustomed to the sensation of ES. For chronic conditions, electrodes are usually placed directly over or along the edges of the painful area.[30] For example, electrodes can be placed on the medial and lateral side of the joint being treated (eg, elbow; **Fig. 5**) or directly on the painful

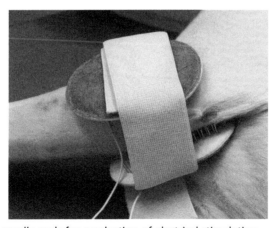

Fig. 4. Brush-like needle pads for conduction of electrical stimulation.

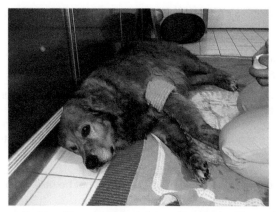

Fig. 5. Electrodes applied to either side of a joint and secured with an elastic strap.

area (eg, back; **Figs. 6** and **7**). The placement of electrodes to the sides of the spine near the nerve origins of the target treatment area is recommended for acute conditions or when direct or more local application of electrodes is not possible. Other possibilities are the placement over acupuncture or trigger points, and along peripheral superficial nerve tracts.

Electrical Stimulation for Pain Control

Several theories explain the pain-relieving mechanisms behind ES: the gate control theory,[31] a release of endogenous opiates,[32–34] an increase in blood flow and reduction in muscle tone,[35] and the counterirritant theory.[36] The term transcutaneous electrical nerve stimulation (TENS) is commonly used to describe a stimulator used for pain control. The conventional TENS (also called sensory-level TENS) uses frequencies ranging from 50 to 150 Hz and a pulse duration of less than 50 microseconds with a low intensity (high-frequency, low-intensity TENS), and is one of the most often used current parameters. This stimulation mode is presumed to stimulate the gate control and counterirritant mechanisms. Low-frequency TENS (also called motor-level TENS) is a low-frequency, high-intensity type of stimulation with frequencies ranging from 1 to 10 Hz and pulse durations ranging from 100 to 600 microseconds,

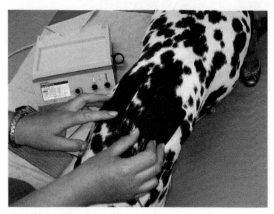

Fig. 6. Electrodes set up for treatment of the back.

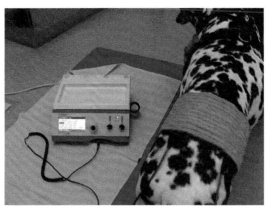

Fig. 7. Electrodes secured to the back with elastic strap.

with a high intensity. Low-frequency TENS is administered at intensities that evoke visible muscle contractions, and is proposed to stimulate the release of endogenous opioids. Regarding this type of stimulation, some investigators differentiate between acupuncture-like TENS with frequencies between 1 and 4 Hz and frequencies between 5 and 10 Hz. These modes may both be applied to acupuncture points or motor points in the segmentally related myotome.[35,36] Another common application is mixed-frequency TENS whereby both sensory and motor-level TENS are applied in the same treatment. The combination of sensory and motor-like TENS is thought to prevent nervous system adaption/accommodation to one particular set of parameters. Varying the TENS parameters (termed modulation) has been shown to prevent accommodation in humans.[37]

Indications for Transcutaneous Electrical Nerve Stimulation

TENS for pain control can be used in numerous orthopedic and neurologic disorders. In humans it has been used for the treatment of acute pain,[38] musculoskeletal pain,[39] and osteoarthritis.[40] In the treatment of musculoskeletal pain, a meta-analysis of existing studies was performed, from which the investigators concluded that high-frequency TENS and TENS with frequencies lower than 10 Hz had a significant effect, whereas acupuncture TENS fell just short of significance.[39] In a meta-analysis study of osteoarthritis of the knee, the combined efficacies of conventional TENS and acupuncture-like TENS were shown to improve pain and stiffness in comparison with placebo treatment. This pain-relieving effect was also found if conventional and acupuncture-like TENS were evaluated separately. Another result of this study was that pain relief by acupuncture-like TENS was approximately 2 times better than that with high frequencies.[40] Rainov and Heidecke[41] investigated the impact of TENS on pain in humans who underwent lumbar canal stenosis surgery. One group of patients received only pain medications and the other group received pain medications and TENS. In the TENS-treated group, the total given dose of medications was significantly reduced in comparison with the control group. Nevertheless, despite the positive results of the experimental research, the use of TENS in clinical practice is debated, as other studies have not shown positive results.[42,43] Unfortunately, few high-quality studies in veterinary medicine are available. In a study of obese dogs suffering from osteoarthritis (OA), a combination of dietary management and intensive physiotherapy including TENS treatments was shown to effectively reduce disability.[44] In a preliminary study, positive effects of TENS application for arthritic pain in the stifle joint of 5 dogs was apparent up to 210 minutes after TENS application, but the greatest improvement was found immediately (first 30 minutes) after treatment.[45] Further study of TENS application in dogs is needed to establish effectiveness. Such studies should include larger groups of animals, different parameters, and altered physical activity throughout the study.

Intensity, Treatment Time, and Frequency of Transcutaneous Electrical Nerve Stimulation

In general, the intensity must always be adapted to the needs, comfort, and response of the individual patient. The recommended intensity varies with the goal of treatment and toleration by the patient. Conventional TENS (high frequency, low intensity) is applied with the intensity of the current just below the sensory response threshold. The intensity is increased until the patient feels a tingling sensation. No muscle contraction should occur. In dogs this can be achieved by carefully increasing of the intensity until the animal shows a reaction such as looking at the pads. For low-frequency TENS, the intensity is slowly increased until the motor threshold is reached, as evidenced by a visible twitch contraction.

In the treatment of humans, various recommendations for treatment time and intervals of the TENS can be found in the literature. For example, in the treatment of OA using conventional TENS, recommended treatment times vary between 15,[44] 30,[45–47] and 60 minutes.[48] The recommended frequency of treatment varies from 3 sessions daily for 3 weeks[48] to twice daily for 6 weeks and up to 2 times per week over 4 weeks.[49] For animals, the following is recommended: lower intensity, short treatment duration, and short intervals between treatment sessions are suitable in acute stages; higher intensities with longer treatment durations and intervals between the treatments are recommended in chronic conditions.[35,36]

Electrical Stimulation for Muscle Strengthening

ES has been used in hundreds of human trials to increase muscle strength. A term commonly associated with ES for muscle strengthening is called neuromuscular electrical stimulation (NMES). NMES has numerous applications for small animals. Examples include patients who have muscle atrophy, in the immediate postoperative period after surgery to manage cranial cruciate ligament injuries, and after femoral head and neck ostectomy. Muscle atrophy seen with nerve injuries, such as radial nerve paralysis, can be attenuated with NMES while waiting for nerve innervation to return. Optimal parameters have not been adequately studied; however, in one trial in dogs with postoperative extracapsular stabilization after cranial cruciate ligament rupture, atrophy was minimized compared with the control group.[50]

Animal Reaction/Safety for Electrical Stimulation

As ES can produce pain if used incorrectly, precautions should be taken to avoid injury to the handler and animal. A muzzle may need to be applied and the animal placed in lateral recumbency during the initial treatment. In some cases, tranquilization may be necessary if the animal is anxious. The authors recommend that treatment only be given under the supervision of trained personnel. Most dogs tolerate ES well, but occasionally a dog may find the sensation unpleasant and vocalize and/or try to run. Turning the current up very slowly is one way to allow the dog to get used to the sensation gradually and tolerate the treatment well.

Types of Stimulators

A large variety of electrical stimulators are commercially available, including small portable units and large units. Some multipurpose units generate ES in a variety of modes and waveforms. These units may also incorporate therapeutic US and/or therapeutic laser.

SUMMARY

PAMs can be effective treatments and/or adjuncts to treatments in the overall rehabilitation plan. Understanding the effects, indications, contraindications, and precautions of each modality is critical for proper use. Selection of the appropriate modality depends largely on an understanding of the diagnosis, an accurate assessment of the stage of tissue healing and repair, an accurate clinical assessment of the functional limitations, the established treatment goals, and continued reevaluation of the patient. Cryotherapy is most useful during the acute inflammatory stages of tissue healing to cause vasoconstriction and to decrease edema and pain. Using heat too soon in the inflammatory process may exacerbate the inflammatory process and slow healing. Heating modalities (both superficial and deep) are most commonly used to cause vasodilation and increase tissue extensibility, and to decrease pain and muscle spasm. ES is most commonly used to reduce pain and muscle spasm, in both acute and chronic circumstances, and to increase muscle strength.

REFERENCES

1. Fruth SJ, Michlovitz SL. Cold therapy. In: Michlovitz SL, Bellew JW, Nolan TP, editors. Modalities for therapeutic intervention. 5th edition. Philadelphia: FA Davis; 2012. p. 21–5.
2. Prentice WE. Cryotherapy and thermotherapy. In: Prentice WE, editor. Therapeutic modalities in rehabilitation. 4th edition. Philadelphia: McGraw-Hill; 2011. p. 285–6.
3. Dragone L, Heinrichs K, Levine D, et al. Superficial thermal modalities. In: Millis D, Levine D, editors. Canine rehabilitation and physical therapy. 2nd edition. Philadelphia: Saunders; 2014. p. 312–27.
4. McMaster WC. A literary review on ice therapy in injuries. Am J Sports Med 1977;5(3):124–6.
5. Knight KL. Cryotherapy in sport injury management. Champaign (IL): Human Kinetics; 1995.
6. Young K, Atherton E. Cryotherapy. In: Shankar K, Randall KD, editors. Therapeutic Physical Modalities. Philadelphia: Hanley & Belfus; 2002. p. 47.
7. Algafly AA, George KP. The effect of cryotherapy on nerve conduction velocity, pain threshold and pain tolerance. Br J Sports Med 2007;41(6):365–9.
8. Millard RP, Towle-Millard HA, Rankin DC, et al. Effect of cold compress application on tissue temperature in healthy dogs. Am J Vet Res 2013;74(3):443–7.
9. Rexing J, Dunning D, Siegel AM, et al. Effects of cold compression, bandaging, and microcurrent electrical therapy after cranial cruciate ligament repair in dogs. Vet Surg 2010;39(1):54–8.
10. Martimbianco AL, Gomes da Silva BN, de Carvalho AP, et al. Effectiveness and safety of cryotherapy after arthroscopic anterior cruciate ligament reconstruction. A systematic review of the literature. Phys Ther Sport 2014. [Epub ahead of print]. http://dx.doi.org/10.1016/j.ptsp.2014.02.008.

11. Drygas KA, McClure SR, Goring RL, et al. Effect of cold compression therapy on postoperative pain, swelling, range of motion, and lameness after tibial plateau leveling osteotomy in dogs. J Am Vet Med Assoc 2011;238(10):1284–91.

12. Price R, Lehmann JF, Boswell-Bessette S, et al. Influence of cryotherapy on spasticity at the human ankle. Arch Phys Med Rehabil 1993;74(3):300–4.

13. Altintas B, Altintas AA, Kraemer R, et al. Acute effects of local cold therapy in superficial burns on pain, in vivo microcirculation, edema formation and histomorphology. Burns 2014;40(5):915–21.

14. Venter TH, Karpelowsky JS, Rode H. Cooling of the burn wound: the ideal temperature of the coolant. Burns 2007;33(7):917–22.

15. Vannetta M, Millis DM, Levine D. The effects of cryotherapy on in-vivo skin and muscle temperature, and intramuscular blood flow. J Orthop Sports Phys Ther 2006;36(1):A47.

16. Okcu G, Yercan HS. Is it possible to decrease skin temperature with ice packs under casts and bandages? A cross-sectional, randomized trial on normal and swollen ankles. Arch Orthop Trauma Surg 2006;126(10):668–73.

17. Weresh MJ, Bennett GL, Njus G. Analysis of cryotherapy penetration: a comparison of the plaster cast, synthetic cast, Ace wrap dressing, and Robert-Jones dressing. Foot Ankle Int 1996;17(1):37–40.

18. Cameron MH. Physical agents in rehabilitation: from research to practice. Philadelphia: Saunders; 1999.

19. Lehmann JF, Masock AJ, Warren CG, et al. Effect of therapeutic temperatures on tendon extensibility. Arch Phys Med Rehabil 1970;51(8):481–7.

20. Levine D, Millis DL, Mynatt T. Effects of 3.3-MHz ultrasound on caudal thigh muscle temperature in dogs. Vet Surg 2001;30(2):170–4.

21. Steiss JE, Adams CC. Effect of coat on rate of temperature increase in muscle during ultrasound treatment of dogs. Am J Vet Res 1999;60(1):76–80.

22. Saini NS, Roy KS, Bansal PS, et al. A preliminary study on the effect of ultrasound therapy on the healing of surgically severed Achilles tendons in five dogs. J Vet Med A Physiol Pathol Clin Med 2002;49(6):321–8.

23. Maia Filho AL, Villaverde AB, Munin E, et al. Comparative study of the topical application of Aloe vera gel, therapeutic ultrasound and phonophoresis on the tissue repair in collagenase-induced rat tendinitis. Ultrasound Med Biol 2010; 36(10):1682–90.

24. Silveira PC, Victor EG, Schefer D, et al. Effects of therapeutic pulsed ultrasound and dimethylsulfoxide (DMSO) phonophoresis on parameters of oxidative stress in traumatized muscle. Ultrasound Med Biol 2010;36(1):44–50.

25. Ng GY, Wong RY. Ultrasound phonophoresis of panax notoginseng improves the strength of repairing ligament: a rat model. Ultrasound Med Biol 2008; 34(12):1919–23.

26. Levine D, Watson T. Therapeutic ultrasound. In: Millis DL, Levine D, editors. Canine rehabilitation and physical therapy. 2nd edition. Philadelphia: Saunders; 2014. p. 328–41.

27. Draper DO, Sunderland S, Kirkendall DT, et al. A comparison of temperature rise in human calf muscles following applications of underwater and topical gel ultrasound. J Orthop Sports Phys Ther 1993;17(5):247–51.

28. Forrest G, Rosen K. Ultrasound: effectiveness of treatments given under water. Arch Phys Med Rehabil 1989;70(1):28–9.

29. Hooker DN, Prentice WE. Basic principles of electricity and electrical stimulating currents. In: Prentice WE, editor. Therapeutic modalities in rehabilitation. 4th edition. Philadelphia: McGraw-Hill; 2011. p. 97–174.

30. Johnson MI, Ashton CH, Thompson JW. The consistency of pulse frequencies and pulse patterns of transcutaneous electrical nerve stimulation (TENS) used by chronic pain patients. Pain 1991;44(3):231–4.
31. Melzack R, Wall PD. Pain mechanisms: a new theory. Science 1965;150(3699): 971–9.
32. Han JS, Chen XH, Sun SL, et al. Effect of low- and high-frequency TENS on Met-enkephalin-Arg-Phe and dynorphin A immunoreactivity in human lumbar CSF. Pain 1991;47(3):295–8.
33. Hughes G, Lichstein P, Whithlock D. Response of plasma betaendorphins to transcutaneous electrical stimulation in healthy subjects. Phys Ther 1984;64: 1062–6.
34. Kalra A, Urban MO, Sluka KA. Blockade of opioid receptors in rostral ventral medulla prevents antihyperalgesia produced by transcutaneous electrical nerve stimulation (TENS). J Pharmacol Exp Ther 2001;298(1):257–63.
35. Bochstahler B, Levine D, Millis DL. Essential facts of physiotherapy in dogs and cats. 1st edition. Babenhausen (Germany): BE VetVerlag; 2004.
36. Levine D, Bochstahler B. Electrical stimulation. In: Millis DL, Levine D, editors. Canine rehabilitation and physical therapy. 2nd edition. Philadelphia: Saunders; 2014. p. 342–58.
37. DeSantana JM, Walsh DM, Vance C, et al. Effectiveness of transcutaneous electrical stimulation for treatment of hyperalgesia and pain. Curr Rheumatol Rep 2008;10(6):492–9.
38. Simpson PM, Fouche PF, Thomas RE, et al. Transcutaneous electrical nerve stimulation for relieving acute pain in the prehospital setting: a systematic review and meta-analysis of randomized-controlled trials. Eur J Emerg Med 2014;21(1):10–7.
39. Johnson M, Martinson M. Efficacy of electrical nerve stimulation for chronic musculoskeletal pain: a meta-analysis of randomized controlled trials. Pain 2007;130(1–2):157–65.
40. Osiri M, Welch V, Brosseau L, et al. Transcutaneous electrical nerve stimulation for knee osteoarthritis. Cochrane Database Syst Rev 2000;(4):CD002823.
41. Rainov N, Heidecke V. Transcutaneous electrical nerve stimulation (TENS) for acute postoperative pain after spinal surgery. Eur J Pain 1994;15:44–9.
42. Albright J, Allmann R, Bonfiglio R. Philadelphia Panel evidence-based clinical practice guidelines on selected rehabilitation interventions for low back pain. Phys Ther 2001;81(10):1641–74.
43. Khadilkar A, Milne S, Brosseau L, et al. Transcutaneous electrical nerve stimulation for the treatment of chronic low back pain: a systematic review. Spine (Phila Pa 1976) 2005;30(23):2657–66.
44. Mlacnik E, Bockstahler B, Muller M, et al. Effects of caloric restriction and a moderate or intense physiotherapy program for treatment of lameness in overweight dogs with osteoarthritis. J Am Vet Med Assoc 2006;229(11):1756–60.
45. Levine D, Johnson K, Price M. The effect of TENS on osteoarthritic pain in the stifle of dogs. In: Proc 2nd Intl Symp Rehabil Phys Therap Vet Med. 2002.
46. Fargas-Babjak A, Rooney P, Gerecz E. Randomized trial of Codetron for pain control in osteoarthritis of the hip/knee. Clin J Pain 1989;5(2):137–41.
47. Grimmer K. A controlled double blind study comparing the effects of strong Burst Mode TENS and High Rate TENS on painful osteoarthritic knees. Aust J Physiother 1992;38(1):49–56.
48. Lewis B, Lewis D, Cumming G. The comparative analgesic efficacy of transcutaneous electrical nerve stimulation and a nonsteroidal anti-inflammatory drug for painful osteoarthritis. Br J Rheumatol 1994;33(5):455–60.

49. Smith CR, Lewith GT, Machin D. TNS and osteo-arthritic pain. Preliminary study to establish a controlled method of assessing transcutaneous nerve stimulation as a treatment for the pain caused by osteo-arthritis of the knee. Physiotherapy 1983;69(8):266–8.
50. Millis DL, Levine D, Weigel JP. A preliminary study of early physical therapy following surgery for cranial cruciate ligament rupture in dogs [abstract]. Vet Surg 1997;26:434.

Therapeutic Laser in Veterinary Medicine

Brian Pryor, PhD[a], Darryl L. Millis, MS, DVM, DACVS, CCRP, DACVSMR[b],*

KEYWORDS

- Laser therapy • Therapeutic laser • Photobiomodulation • Veterinary laser treatment

KEY POINTS

- Laser therapy is an increasingly studied modality that can be a valuable tool for veterinary practitioners to successfully treat conditions whether in a rehabilitation clinic or in a general practice.
- Understanding the basics of light penetration into tissue allows evaluation of the correct dosage to deliver for the appropriate condition, as well as for a particular patient, based on physical properties.
- Photobiomodulation has several potential benefits and using this technology in a systematic way may allow for the discovery of other applications.
- New applications are currently being studied for some of the most challenging health conditions and this field will continue to grow as we learn more.
- Additional clinical studies are still needed and collaboration is highly encouraged for all practitioners using this technology.

Laser therapy is rapidly becoming a modality that is used in a variety of conditions in veterinary medicine. It is estimated that close to 20% of veterinary hospitals in North America are using a therapeutic laser in their practice. Although lasers have been used for many years, it has been only in the past 5 or 6 years that use of laser therapy has become so widespread. The main reasons for this recent change are as follows: an increased awareness and deployment of veterinary rehabilitation services, availability of educational resources on therapy lasers, and the development of products and protocols that have resulted in more consistent clinical outcomes. Because laser therapy is a noninvasive, drug-free treatment option, many clients are happy with a nonpharmacologic treatment option.

Research in the area of photobiomodulation is continuing to increase. Many studies are now focused on particular conditions with translational studies from the laboratory to the clinic. Understanding the basics will allow the therapist to

[a] LiteCure LLC, 250 Corporate Boulevard, Suite 8, Newark, DE 19702, USA; [b] Department of Small Animal Clinical Sciences, College of Veterinary Medicine, University of Tennessee, 2407 River Drive, Knoxville, TN 37996, USA
* Corresponding author.
E-mail address: dmillis@utk.edu

Vet Clin Small Anim 45 (2015) 45–56
http://dx.doi.org/10.1016/j.cvsm.2014.09.003   vetsmall.theclinics.com
0195-5616/15/$ – see front matter © 2015 Published by Elsevier Inc.

accurately prescribe this modality for appropriate conditions in the practice whether it be the main treatment option or as an important adjunctive to other treatments.

THE BASICS

When laser light is absorbed by a chromophore, a biochemical change can occur. There are several examples in nature where this happens, including photosynthesis or the production of vitamin D via conversion by sunlight. Laser therapy or photobiomodulation, the scientific term for this phenomenon is an example of a photochemical process in which light from a laser, or other light source, interacts with cells and causes stimulation or other biochemical change. The term photobiomodulation is most appropriate, as some biochemical events are upregulated and others can be downregulated. Other terms that have been used are cold laser therapy (not accurate, as there is often heat produced during clinical treatments), low-level laser therapy, low light therapy, or nonablative laser therapy, which separates this treatment from more invasive laser surgical procedures. There are many published studies regarding photobiomodulation. A large number of these studies have been performed on cells in vitro. There are excellent published studies on light's effects on various types of cells. Increases in angiogenesis,[1,2] neurite extension,[3] normalization of ion channels,[4] stabilization of the cellular membrane,[5] and a host of other cellular changes have been investigated and published.

The mechanism of action associated with photobiomodulation is often still questioned among scientists in the field. There are most likely several mechanisms of action depending on the target and the type of cell being modulated. The most published and recognized mechanism is that of the cytochrome c system, which is found in the inner cell membrane in the mitochondria and acts as a photoreceptor. Cytochrome c absorbs light from 500 to 1100 nm due to specific properties of this large molecule.[6] After laser light is absorbed by cytochrome c, it is excited and breaks bonds with nitric oxide (NO). This action allows bonding with oxygen to become more prevalent and cytochrome c oxidase to be produced at an optimal rate. Cytochrome c oxidase is critical to the formation of ATP. ATP is essential for energy production in the cell and results in many favorable biologic responses or secondary mechanisms, including reduction of pain and inflammation, and tissue healing.

REDUCING PAIN

There have been extensive studies evaluating various mechanisms of photobiomodulation that may result in pain relief.[7,8] On laser interaction with cells, the following processes may occur:

- Increase in serotonin (5-HT) levels[9-11]
- Increase in beta endorphins,[12-14] whose reception reduces the sensation of pain.
- Increase in NO,[15] which has an effect on vasodilatation and may enhance oxygen delivery.
- Decreases bradykinins[16]; bradykinins normally induce pain sensation by stimulating nociceptive afferent nerves
- Normalization of ion channels[4,17]
- Block depolarization of C-fiber afferent nerves[18]
- Increase nerve cell action potential[19]
- Improve axonal sprouting and nerve cell regeneration[3,20-22]

REDUCING INFLAMMATION

In addition to the previously described mechanisms for reducing pain, laser treatments may reduce inflammation. The following actions may produce key elements that aid in the reduction of edema and inflammation. The following processes may be enhanced:

- ATP production[23,24]
- Stimulation of vasodilatation by induction of NO[25]
- Reduction of interleukin-1[26]
- Stabilization of cellular membranes[5]
- Acceleration of leukocyte activity[27]
- Decrease in prostaglandin, synthesis[28,29]
- Lymphocyte response[30]
- Angiogenesis[1,2]
- Superoxide dismutase (SOD) levels[31,32]

PROMOTING HEALING

Wound healing is the area in which most of the traditional laser therapeutic studies have been completed. The results of these studies have been very encouraging and the mechanisms of tissue healing are important for other injuries, such as tears and contusions of muscles, tendons, and ligaments, as many of the same mechanisms are needed to promote healing in all tissues. The following is a list of important physiologic changes with laser treatment:

- Enhanced leukocyte infiltration[30]
- Increased macrophage activity[33–35]
- Increased neovascularization[36]
- Increased fibroblast proliferation[37,38]
- Keratinocyte proliferation[39]
- Early epithelialization[40]
- Increased growth factors[41,42]
- Greater wound tensile strength[43]

HOW DOES LIGHT PENETRATE? WHAT DOSAGES ARE NEEDED?

Wavelengths in the range from the blue (400 nm) to the mid infrared (1100 nm) can result in a photochemical change in cells.[6] Light-tissue interaction is critical to understand how light penetrates biologic tissue to deliver the appropriate amount of light to the target tissue. When reviewing published studies, you should note whether the study was done in vivo or in vitro. Also notice the type and size of the animal used in the study. Dosages used in culture will be vastly different from those used to treat a laboratory rodent. Dosages needed in a clinical environment also differ regarding patient size, with much greater doses needed for treating a Siberian husky compared to a feline patient.

Depth of penetration is one of the most critical elements of laser treatment. When light interacts with biological tissue, it is absorbed, scattered (including reflection), and/or transmitted. Wavelengths from 600 nm (red end of the spectrum) to 1100 nm (near infrared end of the spectrum) are in the optimal range for penetrating into tissue (**Fig. 1**). This range of wavelengths is often referred to as the "therapeutic window" for light and laser applications. Although these wavelengths are able to penetrate, each wavelength has unique properties and each will penetrate to different depths. When white light is placed on tissue, like a flashlight in your mouth, we will see red light

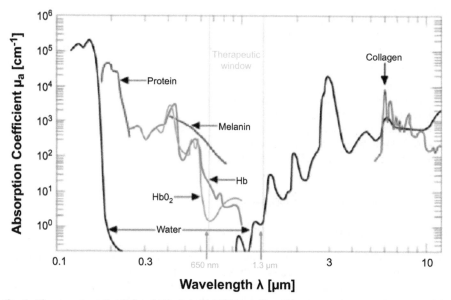

Fig. 1. The wavelength of the photons is important in laser therapy. Various substances preferentially absorb laser light at different wavelengths. (*From* Millis DL, Gross Saunders D. Laser therapy in canine rehabilitation. In: Millis DL, Levine D, editors. Canine rehabilitation and physical therapy. Philadelphia: Elsevier; 2014. p. 361 with permission.)

coming through because the blue and, to some extent, the red components are absorbed, mostly by hemoglobin. A general rule is that longer wavelengths penetrate deeper into tissue.

The major chromophores that absorb light and prevent light penetration to target tissues are melanin, hemoglobin, and water. Melanin has a very high absorption, so dark skin absorbs more light, especially for wavelengths less than 830 nm. Wavelengths longer than 1300 nm absorb strongly in water and therefore penetration is difficult. Light from longer-wavelength lasers, such as the CO_2 laser that operates at 10,600 nm, is absorbed strongly by water and is consequently used for surgical applications.[44]

The important parameter for a therapy laser system is to have the appropriate wavelength to allow penetration to deep tissue. Wavelengths longer than 800 nm can typically achieve appropriate depths to treat most musculoskeletal conditions. When dealing with wounds or more superficial conditions, shorter wavelengths, such as 635 nm, can be used effectively, because penetration is less important.

A recent nerve repair study demonstrated that 2.45% of the initial light at 980 nm penetrated to the peroneal nerve on an anesthetized large New Zealand white rabbit, through approximately 3 cm of tissue. The laser was delivered directly to the skin and a specialty power meter was inserted under the muscle directly on top of the nerve. The percentage of light penetrating to the nerve was constant with increased laser power. This experiment also yielded a similar percentage of transmitted light when using 810-nm or 980-nm light.[22]

Because light from all wavelengths has a measurable amount of scatter, absorption, or transmission, the more power, or the greater number of photons delivered, the greater depth of penetration will be achieved as a function of time. For example, assume that 2.5% of the initial light delivered to the skin reaches the hip of a small dog. Using a 300-mW output laser, 7.5 mW of light will reach the joint space, or just

0.0075 J per second of treatment time. Using a higher-power laser will result in proportionally higher energy delivered to the joint. Lower-powered lasers must be used for longer times to achieve a large enough dose to be effective. It has been shown that extremely low exposures, less than 0.100 mW/cm^2, even when exposed for a long period of time, have no measurable results.[45]

Dosage can be expressed only as the amount of energy delivered to a certain area on the surface. Penetration work using cadavers and laboratory animals, as well as extrapolation from tissue studies has increased our understanding of the amount of light delivered to various target tissue depths. Dosages from 2 to 20 J/cm^2 applied to the surface appear to be an appropriate range for photobiomodulation. The patient's size, body type, coat color, skin color, coat length, and the depth of the condition are the important parameters needed to calculate the correct dosage. The larger the dog, the larger the dosage needed.

The treatment of most deep musculoskeletal conditions for a medium-size dog requires 4 to 8 J/cm^2. If the dog is thin, clipped, and has a light-colored coat and skin, the dosage may be at the lower end at 4 J/cm^2. Larger body types require higher dosages because there is more tissue to penetrate through. When treating a surface contusion, 2 to 3 J/cm^2 is an adequate dose because penetration is not as essential due to the superficial nature of the injury.

APPLICATIONS FOR LASER THERAPY
Rehabilitation Applications

Lasers are very commonly found in many rehabilitation practices. They are used as an integral part of rehabilitation protocols. It is important to use laser therapy appropriately in conjunction with surgical interventions, other modalities, exercise, massage, and pharmacologic options. Often the laser gives patients enough comfort to allow patients to initiate or increase certain exercise protocols, such as increasing range of motion of a stiff joint. Here are some common rehabilitation applications:

- Postsurgical treatment: edema control and healing
- Nonoperative muscle, ligament, tendon injury: pain management and reducing inflammation, potential improved healing depending on the size and nature of the injury (**Fig. 2**)
- Muscle, ligament, tendon strains and sprains: reduction of pain and inflammation, improved healing times
- Nerve damage: nerve regrowth, pain management
- Arthritis: reduction of pain and inflammation

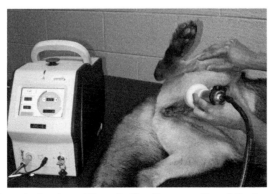

Fig. 2. Laser treatment of a dog with early fibrotic myopathy of the inner thigh muscles.

General Practice Applications

- Otitis: an adjunctive therapy used for reducing inflammation in the ear, possibly allowing for better penetration of medication and better compliance
- Lick granulomas: treatment may improve healing rates, as well as remove the irritation leading to less self-trauma. Treat with higher dosages than a standard wound. The suggested dosage should be 15 to 20 J/cm^2
- Postsurgical incisions: treatment for pain as well as healing, less scarring of incisions
- Wounds: improved healing times and less scarring
- Arthritis: management of pain and reduce inflammation, routine maintenance is required
- Inflammatory conditions: lessen pain, and reduce edema

TREATMENT TECHNIQUES

Treatment techniques vary depending on the condition being treated and the type of laser being used. As previously discussed regarding dosing, when treating a condition in deeper tissues, a greater dose will be required.

Prepare the surface. Make sure the hair/skin is clean. Clipping the hair is optimal for the best penetration of light into the tissue. If the hair is not clipped, be sure to increase the dosage to allow enough light to penetrate into the tissue, although studies are needed to determine the amount of increased dose. Hair and skin color are important because light of shorter wavelengths is absorbed more by melanin. Some commercially available therapeutic lasers vary wavelengths based on coat and skin color. If wavelengths less than 900 nm are used, be cautious not to overheat the coat or skin if higher power (Watts) is used. Lower the output power and treat with a greater dosage to deliver enough energy to the targeted tissue. If an overweight patient is being treated in an area with increased tissue thickness, be sure to increase the dosage because more light will be absorbed by tissues.

It is often difficult to isolate a very specific afflicted area, and often conditions will have multiple involved muscles or joints contributing to the pain. It is wise to have a broad area of treatment. Cover a large comprehensive area with the appropriate dosage. This enables the affected area and satellite areas of pain to be effectively treated. Treating a comprehensive area will ensure more consistent outcomes, as well as easier protocols for technicians to follow.

When treating there are 2 treatment techniques. Lower-power laser systems, less than 1 Watt, generally use a point-to-point method of treatment. Multiple discrete points are treated in the desired area. The dosage at each spot is delivered in approximately 30 seconds depending on the power and spot size. This method can be very time consuming when treating a large area and does not lend itself well to efficient treatment of multiple areas.

The second technique is to move the laser in a scanning fashion while treating. This method is used when using a higher-output powered laser. The dosage is delivered over a very large area by scanning the laser over the area. This technique allows for comprehensive coverage allowing for multiple areas to be treated. Most higher-power lasers have larger spot sizes, making the power density safer. Caution should always be exercised by realizing the power density and ensure the laser handpiece is moving during treatment.

When treating, the laser can also be applied in a contact or an off-contact mode. By using on-contact mode, the soft tissues may be manipulated while delivering the treatment. This allows deeper treatment because of tissue compression, and, if desired, a gentle massage is administered while delivering the light. Patients seem to enjoy this contact method. When touching the surface is undesirable because of excessive pain, a bony prominence, or a wound, use an off-contact method. In this case, the laser handpiece is kept above the surface during treatment.

Positioning the patient is important before administration of the therapy. Make sure the patient is comfortable and that you have access to the treatment area. When possible, it is also good technique to try to put the body part being treated through some limited, passive range of motion. Be as comprehensive as possible, treating from as many sides as possible.

The frequency of the treatments somewhat depends on the nature of the condition and access to the patient. It is acceptable to treat every day. When treating an acute injury, treatment every day is ideal. It you cannot have access to the patient every day, treat as often as you can see the patient. For more chronic conditions, initial treatments can be administered every other day. The initial phase of treatments should be done until a noticeable result is seen. This change is typically achieved earlier for acute conditions (2 or 3 treatments) than with more chronic conditions (4–6 treatments). The next treatment phase can space treatments out to 2 or 3 treatments per week until healing or the desired effect is achieved. Treatment is then given on an as-needed maintenance schedule depending on the condition of the patient.

PRACTICE INTEGRATION

Adding any new treatment option into a practice can be an exciting and rewarding experience, but also may cause reservations among some staff members. Staff members should be educated that there is scientific evidence behind the use of therapeutic lasers. Getting the staff to confidently use and prescribe laser therapy is key to fully integrating this modality into the practice. After each person has treated a few cases, confidence increases and it may be one of the most popular treatment options.

An easy way to start integrating laser therapy into your practice is to treat all post-surgical incisions. Laser therapy is indicated for pain relief and wound healing. Because of the superficial nature of this wound, the dosage will be low (typically 2–4 J/cm^2), so the treatment times will be only a few minutes. The treatments can be done while in the operating room or shortly after the surgery. Scheduling is easy because it can be included after every surgery performed in the practice. The typical fee for this service commonly ranges from $10 to $25, but generally the surgical fees are increased by this amount to integrate this new high technology for healing and pain management.

This integration into surgical procedures allows the staff to become familiar with the operation of the laser and increase their confidence level. The next step is to incorporate it into everyday treatments for conditions requiring the reduction of pain and inflammation, as well as healing. Education of all the veterinarians in the practice is key so they are aware of the large number of conditions in which the laser is a treatment option.

Many practices have designated 1 or 2 as laser specialists in the practice. These staff members, usually skilled technicians, can be the primary operators of the therapeutic laser in the clinic. The veterinarians can prescribe laser therapy treatments and the laser technicians can consult and perform the therapy for conditions seen in the general practice. This approach makes scheduling easy and the procedures are efficient for the entire practice.

In a rehabilitation practice, laser therapy is generally used in conjunction with other rehabilitation modalities, such as electrical stimulation. It is used postoperatively not only for pain and wound healing, but also for reducing edema and increasing range of motion. Laser therapy allows the physical therapist to start exercise earlier if the pain level is decreased and the patient is comfortable. Almost every rehabilitation case may be a candidate for using the laser in some manner. Pricing is usually incorporated into a rehabilitation visit. If laser is an add-on modality, prices may range from $30 to $60 per visit. If multiple body parts are treated, a nominal charge may be added on a per-area basis.

In general, an arthritis management program is an excellent addition to any practice. When incorporating physical rehabilitation into an arthritis management program, including laser therapy, results are generally enhanced. Laser may be especially useful to reduce inflammation and manage the pain associated with osteoarthritis.

CLIENT CONSULTS

Laser therapy can often be a difficult treatment modality to explain to a client. Many people have experience themselves with a laser treatment, either for a cosmetic procedure, such as hair removal, or for a surgical procedure, such as corrective eye surgery. It is important to explain the difference that therapeutic laser treatments are nonablative, unlike some of the more invasive laser procedures available in human medicine. During a therapeutic laser treatment, there may be some mild heating but when used appropriately, it does not cause any pain and often can be quite soothing to the animal when used correctly. The Food and Drug Administration has cleared laser therapeutic devices for the indications of wound healing, pain reduction, reduction of inflammation, and increased microcirculation. It is also good to explain that this modality is being used worldwide for many conditions and most professional sports teams are using laser therapy in the locker room, keeping players in the game.

The following is a good layman's explanation of how therapeutic lasers work: The light generated by the laser is activating the body's cells to produce energy. When the cells are injured the energy production in a cell is impaired and often cannot make energy at an optimal rate, which is necessary for tissue to heal. The laser light stimulates this process, which causes the cell to produce more energy leading to faster healing.

Setting expectations of the outcomes is important. For acute conditions, the pain and inflammation may be reduced even after the initial treatment; however, more treatments are usually needed for the best outcomes. For more chronic conditions, such as arthritis, prepare the owner that improvements in their pet's condition may not be noticed until the third or fourth treatment and 10 or more treatment sessions may be needed. In a case like arthritis, the laser is only helping to control inflammation. It will not resolve the condition, but it can be a part of the long-term treatment plan in managing the disease. It is important to explain to clients that routine treatments may be needed to control inflammation and pain. The frequency of these maintenance treatments depends on the pain level and activity level of the animal. Typically treatments may be required every 6 to 8 weeks.

PRECAUTIONS

1. Use protective eye wear (**Fig. 3**). Laser goggles should be matched with the particular laser equipment. Because the eye wear is wavelength-dependent, be sure to use the goggles provided with the laser being used. Specific laser protective eyewear for animals also is available. The patient's eyes can also be directed away from the treatment area or shielded with a dark cloth.

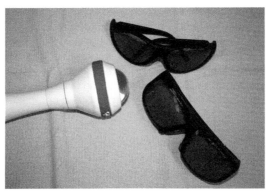

Fig. 3. Protective eyewear for laser use should be specific for the laser used. (*From* Millis DL, Gross Saunders D. Laser therapy in canine rehabilitation. In: Millis DL, Levine D, editors. Canine rehabilitation and physical therapy. Philadelphia: Elsevier; 2014. p. 359–80; with permission.)

2. Use caution when treating dark-colored skin and/or hair, or over tattoos, because more light will be absorbed and potentially heat the tissues more. Use your hand to monitor the skin temperature throughout the treatment, move the laser when using a high-power laser, and if the patient seems uncomfortable, pause the treatment.
3. Do not direct the laser into the eye.
4. Treatment is not recommended over open fontanels, a pregnant uterus, malignancies, or for patients on photosensitive medications.
5. Remove any jewelry, leashes, and so forth.
6. Use caution around metal surfaces because light will reflect. Cover metal examination tables or other shiny objects.

SUMMARY

Laser therapy is an increasingly studied modality that can be a valuable tool for veterinary practitioners to successfully treat conditions, whether in a rehabilitation clinic or in a general practice. Mechanisms of action have been studied and identified for the reduction of pain and inflammation, as well as the healing of tissue. Understanding the basics of light penetration into tissue allows evaluation of the correct dosage to deliver for the appropriate condition, as well as for a particular patient based on physical properties. Photobiomodulation has several potential benefits and using this technology in a systematic way may allow for the discovery of other applications. New applications are currently being studied for some of the most challenging health conditions and this field will continue to grow as we learn more. Additional clinical studies are needed and collaboration is highly encouraged for all practitioners using this technology. There are a growing number of educational resources about therapeutic lasers and recent advances.

REFERENCES

1. Mirsky N, Krispel Y, Shoshany Y, et al. Promotion of angiogenesis by low energy laser irradiation. Antioxid Redox Signal 2002;4(5):785–90.
2. Bibikova A, Belkin V, Oron U. Enhancement of angiogenesis in regenerating gastrocnemius muscle of the toad (*Bufo viridis*) by low-energy laser irradiation. Anat Embryol (Berl) 1994;190:597–602.

3. Anders JJ, Borke RC, Woolery SK, et al. Low power laser irradiation alters the rate of regeneration of the rat facial nerve. Lasers Surg Med 1993;13(1):72–82.

4. Granados-Soto V, Arguelles CF, Alvarez-Leefmans FJ. Peripheral and central anti-nociceptive action of Na+-K+-2Cl- co-transporter blockers on formalin-induced nociception in rats. Pain 2005;114(1–2):231–8.

5. Greco M, Vacca RA, Moro L, et al. Helium-neon laser irradiation of hepatocytes can trigger increase of the mitochondrial membrane potential and can stimulate c-fos expression in a Ca2+-dependent manner. Lasers Surg Med 2001;29(5):433–41.

6. Karu T. Mechanisms of interaction of monochromatic visible light with cells. Proc SPIE 1995;2630:2–9.

7. Tuner J, Hode L. The laser therapy handbook. Grangeberg (Sweden): Prima Books AB; 2007. p. 68.

8. Pozza D, Fregapani P, Weber J, et al. Analgesic action of laser therapy (LLLT) in an animal model. Med Oral Patol Oral Cir Bucal 2008;13(10):E648–52.

9. Cassone MC, Lombard A, Rossetti V, et al. Effect of in vivo HeNe laser irradiation on biogenic amine levels in rat brains. J Photochem Photobiol B, Biol 1993;18(2–3):291–4.

10. Walker JB. Relief from chronic pain by low-power laser irradiation. Neurosci Lett 1983;43:339–44.

11. Lombard A, Rossetti V, Cassone MC. Neurotransmitter content and enzyme activity variations in rat brain following in vivo HeNe laser irradiation. Proceedings, round table on basic and applied research on photobiology and photomedicine. Bari, Italy, November 10–11, 1990.

12. Montesinos M. Experimental effects of low power laser in encephalin and endorphin synthesis. LASER J Eur Med Laser Assoc 1988;1(3):2–7.

13. Labajos M. Beta-endorphin levels modification after GaAs and HeNe laser irradiation on the rabbit. Comparative study. Invest Clin 1988;1-2:6–8.

14. Laakso EL, Cramond T, Richardson C, et al. ACTH and beta-endorphin levels in response to low level laser therapy for myofascial trigger points. Laser Ther 1994;6(3):133–42.

15. Mrowiec J. Analgesic effect of low-power infrared laser radiation in rats. Proc SPIE 1997;3198:83–9.

16. Jimbo K, Noda K, Suzuki K, et al. Suppressive effects of low-power laser irradiation on bradykinin evoked action potentials in cultured murine dorsal root ganglion cells. Neurosci Lett 1998;240(2):93–6.

17. Friedman H, Lubart R. Nonlinear photobiostimulation: the mechanism of visible and infrared laser-induced stimulation and reduction of neural excitability and growth. Laser Ther 1911;3(1):15–8.

18. Wakabayashi H. Effect of irradiation by semiconductor laser on responses evoked in trigeminal caudal neurons by tooth pulp stimulation. Lasers Surg Med 1993;13(6):605–10.

19. Cambier D, Blom K, Witvrouw E, et al. The influence of low intensity infrared laser irradiation on conduction characteristics of peripheral nerve: a randomised, controlled, double blind study on the sural nerve. Lasers Med Sci 2000;15(3):195–200.

20. Rochkind S, El-Ani D, Nevo Z, et al. Increase of neuronal sprouting and migration using 780nm laser phototherapy as procedure for cell therapy. Lasers Surg Med 2009;41:277–81.

21. Byrnes K, Wu X, Waynant R, et al. Low power laser irradiation alters gene expression of olfactory ensheathing cells in vitro. Lasers Surg Med 2005;37:161–71.

22. Anders JJ, Moges H, Wu X, et al. In vitro and in vivo optimization of infrared laser treatment for injured peripheral nerves. Lasers Surg Med 2014;46:34–5.

23. Mochizuki ON, Kataoka Y, Cui Y. Effects of near-infra-red laser irradiation on adenosine triphosphate and adenosine diphosphate contents in rat brain tissue. Neurosci Lett 2002;323(3):207–10.

24. Passarella S, Casamassima E, Molinari S, et al. Increase of proton electrochemical potential and ATP synthesis in rat liver mitochondria irradiated in vitro by helium-neon laser. FEBS Lett 1984;175:95–9.

25. Shiva S, Gladwin MT. Shining a light on tissue NO stores: near infrared release of NO from nitrite and nitrosylated hemes. J Mol Cell Cardiol 2009;46:1–3.

26. Lopes-Martins RA, Albertini R, Martins PS, et al. Spontaneous effects of low-level laser therapy (650 nm) in acute inflammatory mouse pleurisy induced by carrageenan. Photomed Laser Surg 2005;23:377–81.

27. Mester E, Nagylucskay S, Waidelich W, et al. Effects of direct laser radiation on human lymphocytes. Arch Dermatol Res 1978;263:241–5.

28. Sakurai Y, Yamaguchi M, Abiko Y. Inhibitory effect of low-level laser irradiation on LPS-stimulated prostaglandin E2 production and cyclooxygenase-2 in human gingival fibroblasts. Eur J Oral Sci 2000;108(1):29–34.

29. Mizutani K, Musya Y, Wakae K, et al. A clinical study on serum prostaglandin E2 with low-level laser therapy. Photomed Laser Surg 2004;22(6):537–9.

30. Karu T. Low-intensity laser light action upon fibroblasts and lymphocytes. In: Ohshiro T, Calderhead RG, editors. Progress in laser therapy. Hoboken, NJ: J. Wiley and Sons; 1991. p. 175–80.

31. Lavi R, Shainberg A, Friedmann H, et al. Low energy visible light induces reactive oxygen species generation and stimulates an increase of intracellular calcium concentration in cardiac cells. J Biol Chem 2003;278:40917–22.

32. Lubart R, Eichler M, Lavi R, et al. Low-energy laser irradiation promotes cellular redox activity. Photomed Laser Surg 2005;23:3–9.

33. Dube A, Bansal H, Gupta PK. Modulation of macrophage structure and function by low level He–Ne laser irradiation. Photochem Photobiol Sci 2003;2:851–5.

34. Zeng H, Qin JZ, Xin H, et al. The activating action of low level helium-neon laser irradiation on macrophages in mouse model. Laser Ther 1992;4:55–8.

35. Young SR, Dyson M, Bolton P. Effect of light on calcium uptake by macrophages. Laser Ther 1990;5:53–7.

36. Maeda T. Histological, thermographic and thermometric study in vivo and excised 830 nm diode laser irradiated rat skin. Laser Ther 1990;2(1):32.

37. Vinck EM, Cagnie BJ, Cornelissen MJ, et al. Increased fibroblast proliferation induced by light emitting diode and low power laser irradiation. Lasers Med Sci 2003;18:95–9.

38. Hawkins D, Abrahamse H. Effect of multiple exposure of low-level laser therapy on the cellular responses of wounded human skin fibroblasts. Photomed Laser Surg 2006;24:705–14.

39. Haas AF, Isseroff RR, Wheeland RG, et al. Low-energy helium-neon laser irradiation increases the motility of cultured human keratinocytes. J Invest Dermatol 1990;94:822–6.

40. Bayat M, Vasheghani M, Razavi N, et al. Effect of low-level laser therapy on the healing of second-degree burns in rats: a histological and microbiological study. J Photochem Photobiol B, Biol 2005;78(2):171–7.

41. Stein A, Benayahu D, Maltz L, et al. Low-level laser irradiation promotes proliferation and differentiation of human osteoblasts in vitro. Photomed Laser Surg 2005;23(2):161–6.

42. Mvula B, Mathope T, Moore T, et al. The effect of low level laser therapy on adult human adipose derived stem cells. Lasers Med Sci 2008;23:277–82.
43. Parizotto NA, Baranauskas V. Structural analysis of collagen fibrils after HeNe laser photostimulated regenerating rat tendon. In: 2nd Congress World Association for laser therapy. Proceedings. Kansas City, September 2–5, 1998. p. 66.
44. Hale GM, Querry MR. Optical constants of water in the 200nm to 200μm wavelength region. Appl Opt 1973;12:555–63.
45. Karu T, Andreichuck T, Ryabykh T. Suppression of human blood chemiluminescence by diode laser irradiation at wavelengths 660, 820, 880 or 950 nm. Laser Ther 1993;5:103.

Principles and Application of Range of Motion and Stretching in Companion Animals

Denis J. Marcellin-Little, DEDV[a],*,
David Levine, PT, PhD, DPT, CCRP, Cert. DN[b]

KEYWORDS

- Dog • Joint motion • Range of motion • Passive range of motion • Stretching
- Flexibility • Contracture

KEY POINTS

- Joint motion is a fundamental aspect of locomotion and activities of daily living.
- Joint motion may be restricted in companion animals after injury, surgery, or as a response to acute or chronic conditions.
- Range of motion and stretching exercises are commonly used in companion animal rehabilitation programs to maintain or improve the motion of musculoskeletal tissues and skin.
- Stretching exercises are a critical aspect of the management of joint contractures and myopathies.

INTRODUCTION

Optimal locomotion and activities of daily living require adequate motion of joints, muscles, tendon, fascia, and skin. The motion of these tissues can be negatively affected by injuries, surgery, and by acute and chronic conditions. Joint motion may be transiently or permanently lost. Range of motion (ROM) and stretching exercises positively affect tissue motion and may prevent future injuries from occurring. This article presents the general principles of ROM and stretching exercises, discusses the pathophysiology of problems negatively affecting tissue motion, and reviews the clinical applications of ROM and stretching exercises in companion animals.

ASSESSMENT OF JOINT MOTION

The appreciation of loss of joint motion requires the assessment of joint motion using a goniometer. Most often, clinicians focus on joint motion in a sagittal plane: flexion and

Disclosure: The authors report no conflict of interest.
[a] Department of Clinical Sciences, College of Veterinary Medicine, North Carolina State University, NCSU CVM VHC #2563, 1052 William Moore Drive, Raleigh, NC 27607-4065, USA;
[b] Department of Physical Therapy, 615 McCallie Avenue, Chattanooga, TN 37403-2598, USA
* Corresponding author.
E-mail address: denis_marcellin@ncsu.edu

extension, because that is the primary motion of joints. The method for measuring flexion and extension using a goniometer has been standardized and validated in dogs and cats.[1–3] In Labrador retrievers, for example, passive joint flexion and extension (ROM) is 32° to 196° (total of 164°) in the carpus, 36° to 165° (129°) in the elbow, 57° to 165° (108°) in the shoulder, 39° to 164° (125°) in the tarsus, 42° to 162° (120°) in the stifle, and 50° to 162° (112°) in the hip joint. Cats have a passive joint flexion and extension (ROM) of 22° to 198° (total of 176°) in the carpus, 22° to 163° (141°) in the elbow, 32° to 163° (131°) in the shoulder, 21° to 167° (146°) in the tarsus, 24° to 164° (140°) in the stifle, and 33° to 164° (131°) in the hip joint. There are some differences in joint motion among dog breeds. For example, compared with Labrador retrievers, German shepherds dog have differences in passive joint flexion and extension for the elbow, shoulder, tarsus, stifle, and hip (ie, all joints except the carpus).[3] German shepherd dogs' joints flex more (~10°) and extend less (~10°) than those of Labrador retrievers but overall their joints have the same ROM. The difference between Labrador retrievers and German shepherds dog is associated with Labradors being more upright than Shepherds when they stand and walk. It is not clear whether the Shepherds' gait is the consequence of their joint motion or whether the joint motion is the consequence of their gait. The gaits of Labrador retrievers and Rottweilers trotting on a treadmill were compared. Minor differences (<9°) in carpal, elbow, tarsal, and stifle motion were identified.[4] Obesity has been shown to alter gait. In a study comparing the trot of lean and obese mixed breed dogs, stance phase ROM was greater in obese dogs than in lean dogs in the shoulder (28° vs 21°), elbow (24° vs 16°), hip (27° vs 23°), and tarsal (39° vs 28°) joints.[5] Swing phase ROM was greater in obese dogs than in lean dogs in the elbow (61° vs 54°) and hip (34° vs 30°) joints. Other dog breeds also can have idiosyncratic joint motion that is the result of anatomic issues. For example, greyhounds seem to have less tarsal flexion than Labrador retrievers. The motion of joints is influenced by muscle mass, particularly when muscles of different limb segments can interfere with joint flexion. For example, dogs with muscular pelvic limbs seem to have less stifle flexion than dogs with slender pelvic limbs, and this may also be the reason why cats seem to be able to flex most joints more than dogs despite having similar extension. Joint motion is also influenced by the shape of limbs. For example, chondrodystrophic dogs with antebrachial angular deformities often lack carpal flexion, even in the absence of radiographic signs of osteoarthritis (OA) in their carpi.[6] Although joint motion is essential to being able to use a limb, some types of joint motion are required for limb use and some are not. As a general rule, the motion that is required for limb use corresponds with the ROM used at the walk and trot, and also the gallop if galloping is part of the dog's activities. At a walk, in a kinematic analysis of Labrador retrievers, the flexion and extension (ROM) of the main limb joints were estimated to be 128° to 238° (110° of ROM) in the carpus, 91° to 146° (54°) in the elbow, 88° to 125° (36°) in the shoulder, 111° to 145° (34°) in the tarsus, 111° to 146° (35°) in the stifle, and 111° to 147° (36°) in the hip joint.[7] To go from sit to stand in the same group of dogs, the motion was 133° to 202° (70° of ROM) for the carpus, 109° to 147° (37°) in the elbow, 91° to 119° (27°) in the shoulder, 95° to 131° (35°) in the tarsus, 46° to 108° (62°) in the stifle, and 49° to 115° (66°) in the hip joint.[7] These flexion values correspond with sitting position and these extension values correspond with a standing position. Measurements of joint motion differ slightly in other studies involving kinematic analysis because of differences in methodology, particularly differences in marker placement.

It is important to put loss of joint motion in perspective because the functional consequences of loss of joint motion vary widely. A dog with a loss of passive joint motion that does not overlap the motion used at a trot is likely to show no sign of lameness.

For example, if a Labrador loses ~40° of flexion in the stifle joint as a result of OA, the passive motion of the joint would change from ~40° (flexion) to 160° (extension) to ~80° and ~160° respectively. Because the ROM at a walk is (~110°–~150°), walking would not be affected by that loss of motion. However, sitting straight would not be possible because it requires ~45° of stifle flexion.

Joints also move in other planes: in the coronal plane (adduction and abduction) and in the transverse plane (internal and external rotation), along the long axis of limbs (distraction), and perpendicular to the long axis of limbs (cranial drawer). These motions are referred to as secondary or ancillary. They have less amplitude (ie, are smaller) and are harder to measure, and therefore the information documenting them is generally lacking. Ancillary joint motion is part of normal locomotion and is important in working and sporting dogs. Each joint has a unique set of passive and active ancillary motions. The carpus has approximately 19° of motion in the coronal plane (varus to valgus) in Labradors retrievers.[1] The carpus also has rotational and translational motion, particularly when flexed. The elbow has ~45° of external rotation (supination). The shoulder is a loose joint that has a high degree of abduction (measured at 33° in a group of dogs).[8] The shoulder also has internal and external rotation, adduction, and it can be distracted, creating cavitation in the joint.[9] The tarsus has a small amount of torsional motion. The stifle has extensive rotational motion (particularly internal rotation), which has been poorly described. The stifle may have some cranial drawer (in the absence of cranial cruciate ligament injury), particularly in skeletally immature dogs. The hip has a large amount of abduction, adduction, and external rotation, which are also poorly documented. In general terms, the loss of ancillary joint motion is less detrimental to limb use than the loss of flexion or extension. For example, stifle internal rotation is eliminated when extracapsular stabilization of the stifle joint is performed in cruciate-deficient dogs and elbow supination is severely restricted in dogs that undergo total elbow replacement.

The gait of patients undergoing these surgeries is altered as a result of loss of ancillary joint motion but they can bear weight appropriately, provided that the joints are stable and pain free. Restriction of ancillary joint motion places abnormal stress on bone-implant interfaces and on adjacent joints but the consequences of abnormal joint motion on adjacent joints are poorly described and may not be particularly severe. The clearest example of disorders of the adjacent joint induced by abnormal joint motion is probably the development of bicipital tenosynovitis as a consequence of loss of elbow flexion secondary to elbow OA. Tenosynovitis could be caused by overuse of the biceps brachii muscle.[10] Surgical procedures that alter joint motion may be best suited for dogs in which functional expectations are more limited (ie, in pet dogs rather than working dogs).

GENERAL PRINCIPLES OF RANGE OF MOTION AND STRETCHING EXERCISES

ROM is influenced by the shape of joints, the joint capsule, ligaments, and periarticular tendons and muscles. ROM is related to flexibility and is affected by activity, body condition, and joint health. ROM exercises are exercises that yield flexion and extension in specific joints. Passive ROM is the motion of joints that is the result of the manipulation of limbs or spine by a caregiver. In the past, clinicians avoided moving joints in the early postoperative period after surgical repair of a fracture, luxation, or joint injury but early mobilization is clearly beneficial and leads to an enhanced recovery.[11] Passive ROM promotes cartilage nutrition, decreases adhesion between tissue planes, decreases edema, and provides pain relief through a gate control mechanism. It improves joint motion and can positively affect tissue healing.[11] Passive ROM is now used extensively in the early postoperative period, until active motion returns, and it is used in chronic conditions. Passive ROM involves gentle, repetitive motion of the joint in its midrange (ie, away from full flexion and extension). In the past, passive ROM in veterinary medicine was limited to home instruction and to activities such as bicycling the limb. The principles and specific techniques of passive ROM are now delivered in a specific manner including the direction of movement, the amount of force or stress applied, the number of repetitions, and the frequency of treatment. To help determine the cause of articular, muscle, or connective tissue restrictions in motion, the examiner assesses the end feel. The end feel is the sensation imparted to the examiner's hands at the end of the ROM of the tissue being examined.[12] The normal end feel for most joints is imparted by the joint capsule and is a reflection of the elasticity of that capsule. Normal and abnormal end feels are described in **Table 1**. If passive ROM is performed too aggressively, it may result in pain, reflex inhibition, tissue damage, delayed use of the limb, and fibrosis of the periarticular tissues. The patient should not experience more than minimal pain during passive ROM. Maximal pain-free passive ROM is performed to stress the tissues but keep them within a physiologic limit. Adequate knowledge of the tissue strength postoperatively or in chronic conditions is a prerequisite to safely performing passive ROM.

When performing passive ROM, the dog should be as comfortable as possible, usually on a comfortable surface in lateral recumbency. Passive ROM may also be performed in a standing position or other functional positions such as lying over a ball, wheelbarrowing, or dancing. In any position, it is essential to maintain comfort of the animal and a stress-free position of affected joints. Individual joints are gently flexed and extended (or abducted/adducted, rotated, depending on the motion desired) through their comfortable ROM. The limb proximal to the joint is stabilized, and the limb below the affected joint is grasped and gently moved. The closer the hands are placed to the joint, the lower the forces that are applied to the joint. Over the course of several seconds, a joint is slowly flexed and extended until the first indication of discomfort, such as tensing the limb, turning the head in recognition, or trying to gently push away is noted. The end of the motion is commonly held for 1 to 2 seconds. The patient should never vocalize in pain or attempt to bite. This movement is

Table 1			
Classification of joint end feels			
Type of End Feel	**Definition**	**Causes**	**Examples**
Capsular	Slight elasticity, rubbery feel	Joint capsule elasticity	Normal tarsal flexion and extension
Firm capsular	Decreased elasticity compared with normal	Periarticular fibrosis	Loss of stifle extension after cranial cruciate ligament rupture
Soft tissue approximation	Soft tissues limiting motion	Normal when muscle bodies contact each other to stop joint motion	Normal stifle flexion
Springy	Increased spring or bounce	Joint mouse	Meniscal tear
Hard	Abrupt bony stop	Bony overgrowth, mature contracture	Mature quadriceps contracture
Empty	End of ROM cannot be reached	Pain	Intra-articular fracture

repeated for 10 to 20 repetitions, depending on the animal's reaction to the motion, 3 to 6 times daily. Flexion may be repeated as many times as indicated before performing extension passive ROM, or flexion and extension may be alternated. It is also common to only work in 1 direction, based on joint limitations. For example, it is common to only perform extension passive ROM (but not flexion) after extracapsular stabilization of a cruciate-deficient stifle or after a femoral head ostectomy.

Active ROM is the voluntary motion of joints during activities. Active ROM may be assisted or unassisted. Assistance may be provided by a sling, exercise band, brace, or other device or may be provided by decreasing the forces traveling through joints when exercising in water.[13] Active ROM occurs during all exercises. Active ROM can be used to stretch joints. Therapeutic exercises are often designed to promote (or avoid) specific joint positions.

Stretching is a form of exercise in which a muscle or muscle group is maximally elongated. Stretching is often combined with passive ROM exercises when joints have stiffness and decreased ROM or when muscles or tendons are tight. Stretching is typically performed after or as a continuation of passive ROM. The joint might be taken through its passive ROM and then held at the end point; the exercise then becomes a stretch. Stretching can be static, dynamic, or ballistic. Static stretching is the sustained elongation of muscle fibers for a brief period of time, generally greater than 10 seconds and less than 1 minute. As in performing passive ROM, the limb proximal to the joint is stabilized, and the limb below the affected joint is grasped and gently moved in the desired direction. Over the course of several seconds, a joint is slowly moved until there is the first indication of discomfort, such as tensing the limb, turning the head in recognition, or trying to gently push away. The stretch is held for 20 to 30 seconds as tolerated, and repeated 5 to 10 times. This may be done from 1 to 5 times daily, based on the need and diagnosis. A skeletally immature dog with a distal femoral physeal fracture may need passive ROM and stretching performed 5 times daily to prevent quadriceps contracture. An older arthritic dog lacking elbow extension may only have passive ROM and stretching performed once daily. Static stretching can be sustained over longer periods of time by use of a splint or brace (**Fig. 1**). Dynamic stretching is stretching performed during an activity. Ballistic stretching is a rapidly bouncing stretch. Ballistic stretching is generally not used in companion animals because animals might find it disturbing.

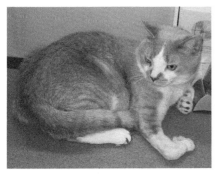 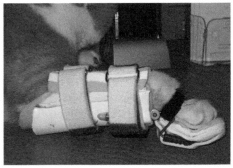

Fig. 1. A cat was rescued and had a lack of carpal extension (*left*). The presence of radial nerve palsy was suspected but an electromyogram indicated that the radial nerve and other nerves were normal. The cat was treated by incorporating a dynamic hinged finger brace (PIP [proximal interphalangeal] Extension Dynasplint system) into a custom splint (*right*).

Stretching is often performed in healthy and athletic dogs as a strategy that could potentially decrease the likelihood of orthopedic injury. After a dog has appropriately warmed up, specific stretches geared toward the type of activity that are planned, or that address preexisting tightness or problem areas in the dog, may be performed. Common areas for stretching include the hips, shoulders, neck, and back muscles. If a dog has sustained an injury that has resulted in residual tightness, such as in an Achilles tendon rupture, stretching of the tight area may reduce the incidence of recurrence, but strengthening exercises combined with stretching provide the best long-term protection against reinjury. To stretch a muscle, it should be placed in a position that produces a slight pull on the muscle but not to the point of pain. With a static stretch, the position in which a slight stretch is felt should be held for 15 to 30 seconds, and each stretch should be repeated 4 to 10 times on each side of the body. The stretch position should not cause pain or take the joint past the normal ROM. The American College of Sports Medicine guidelines are to stretch more than 2 days per week. If the patient has lost some joint motion or feels stiff, ROM or stretching activities should be done daily. However, it is unclear whether stretching has a protective effect with regard to orthopedic injuries during sporting activities in dogs or people and whether it improves performance.[14] Stretching that is too vigorous or performed before warming up can cause injury.

Stretching is also performed in patients that are lacking joint motion as a result of injury or surgery, or in patients with chronic conditions (OA, contractures). As mentioned earlier, not all loss of joint motion has a clinical impact. Stretching is based on the anticipated progression and the clinical impact of loss of joint motion rather than the raw number of degrees lost. A loss of stifle joint flexion after a femoral fracture warrants immediate attention because of the risk of quadriceps contracture. Skeletally immature dogs with distal humeral fractures similarly warrant attention because puppies are at increased risk of loss of joint motion after surgery and the elbow is at increased risk of loss of motion after surgery. With regard to the clinical impact of loss of joint motion, a loss of elbow extension of 10° has a larger clinical impact than a loss of elbow flexion of 40°. Joint motion required to trot comfortably is more clinically important than joint motion beyond the ROM used at a trot. Stretching can be done manually, using external coaptation, or using therapeutic exercises. When planning a stretching program, the clinician in charge should always select the most convenient and least costly method that is likely to succeed. Therapeutic exercises are more convenient than manual therapy but they can only be considered if an effective stretch can be created during exercise. Effective stretches require active joint motion and weight bearing. It is likely that all physical activities have a stretching role on muscles. For example, greyhounds that race have more hip extension than greyhounds that do not race.[15]

When stretching cannot be performed using exercises, coaptation is considered. Low-torque, long-duration stretching is safe and effective.[16] External coaptation can be used to stretch joints that lack motion. Stretching using coaptation is most effective in distal joints (carpus [see **Figs. 1** and **7**] and tarsus) because of thin soft tissue coverage. Stretching using coaptation is possible, but more challenging, in the elbow and stifle. It is not practical for the shoulder and hip joints. A thermomoldable or malleable splint can be used. The splint is shaped so that a gentle sustained stretch is placed on the joint once the leg is wrapped. Dynamic (spring-loaded) hinges or neutral hinges combined with elastic bands are more effective and convenient methods to provide sustained stretch. With dynamic hinges, the torque placed on the joint is often adjustable. That torque is increased over time during the treatment period.

If coaptation is not possible, manual therapy is selected. Manual therapy is the most labor-intensive, and therefore expensive, stretching method. A manual stretching program usually involves 2 to 3 daily stretching sessions for a period of weeks. Whenever possible, joints should be heated for a few (eg, 5 to 10) minutes before and during stretching. A temperature increase of 3 to 4°C is optimal. Stretching heated tissue maximizes safety and effectiveness.[17] Tissue heating is achieved by use of moist heat packs for superficial joints whose depth is less than 3 cm and by use of therapeutic ultrasonography for tissue depths ranging from 3 to 5 cm. The joint torque applied during stretching is adapted to the situation. A weak surgical repair in a young patient in the immediate postoperative period requires a small amount of torque applied often (**Fig. 2**). A chronic situation in a large skeletally mature patient requires preheating and maximal torque (**Fig. 3**). The anticipated gain in joint motion that results from a stretching program is 5 to 10° per week in acute and subacute situations and 3 to 5° per week in chronic situations. Gains are generally more rapid in the early part of the program compared with the late part of the program. Stretching should ideally be taught to patients (so that they tolerate it) and taught to owners (so they perform it safely and effectively) but many patients and owners are not willing or able to perform sustained stretching programs.

Careful documentation of ROM, recorded using goniometry, is necessary to assess problems and monitor their progression and response to therapy. When assessing joint motion, the feel of the joint in full flexion and extension (the end feel) should also be assessed and recorded (see **Table 1**).[12] Firm and hard end feels indicate that the loss of motion is chronic and therefore more difficult to manage.

PATHOPHYSIOLOGY OF JOINT MOTION IN COMPANION ANIMALS

Joint motion may be decreased or increased to the point of interfering with limb use. Loss of joint motion is more common than excess in joint motion. The most common source of loss of joint motion is joint disease, particularly OA. With OA, some joints lose flexion and extension. Subjectively, the motion that is lost is motion that is not

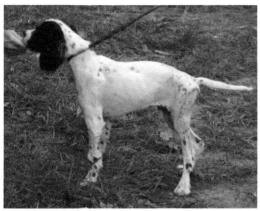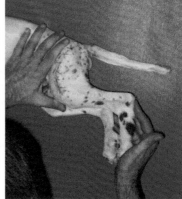

Fig. 2. A 20-week-old English setter sustained a Salter-Harris type II distal femoral fracture that was stabilized using 4 Kirschner wires placed in cross-pin fashion. The day after surgery, the dog holds his stifle joint in extension and has no active stifle joint motion (*left*). Because of the fear of quadriceps contracture, the dog remains hospitalized in a rehabilitation service for an additional week. In the first few days, low-torque stretching of the stifle is performed hourly for a few minutes (*right*).

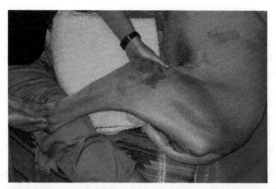

Fig. 3. A 4-year-old Great Dane lost stifle joint extension as a result of a cranial cruciate ligament rupture that was managed without surgery. The dog is mostly non–weight bearing. Stretching sessions, performed twice daily, include preheating the joint with therapeutic ultrasound immediately followed by vigorous stretching.

used during locomotion. For example, elbow OA seems to yield more loss of elbow flexion compared with elbow extension (Marcellin-Little, unpublished data, 2004), possibly because elbow extension is used during the walk and trot (leading dogs to stretch their arthritic elbows when they move) but flexion is not. The loss of ROM secondary to OA rarely has significant clinical consequences, even if it makes the dog's gait stiff or stilted. In a study assessing hip joint motion in Labrador retrievers with hip OA, the mean loss of hip extension was 1° per year.[18] However, some dogs in that study lost up to 40° of hip extension overall. Loss of joint motion also occurs as a result of the occurrence and surgical repair of articular or juxta-articular fractures. This loss of motion may be caused in part by OA being common (70 to 85%) after the repair of an articular fracture in dogs. Also, and more importantly, that loss of motion is caused by periarticular fibrosis, loss of motion between periarticular tissue planes, and the potential development of tethers that connect the fractured region to surrounding muscles. Patients that are skeletally immature seem more likely to lose joint motion after surgery than skeletally mature dogs. Subjectively, hinged joints (eg, elbow, tarsus) are more likely to lose joint motion after juxta-articular surgery than loose joints (eg, shoulder, hip), possibly because hinged joints are tighter and have fewer ancillary joint motions. Dogs undergoing tibial plateau leveling osteotomy (TPLO), a surgery that includes an iatrogenic juxta-articular fracture and its immediate stabilization, have minor changes in stifle joint motion. In one study, mean stifle flexion in patients after TPLO was 37° compared with 29° in controls (unoperated normal contralateral stifles) and mean extension was 155° compared with 160°.[19] Loss of ROM also occurs after joint immobilization because of enzymatic changes in the joint capsule and increase in the number of myofibrobasts on the flexor side of the joint. Joint immobilization is clearly detrimental to musculoskeletal tissues. A complete review of immobilization and remobilization is beyond the scope of this article and is available elsewhere.[20]

The most dramatic form of loss of motion is quadriceps contracture, which can develop a few days to a few weeks after the repair of a femoral fracture, particularly in skeletally immature dogs and cats. In one report describing the management of femoral fractures in 28 cats, 4 cats lost stifle joint motion after surgery (**Fig. 4**).[21] The problem was referred to in the past as fracture disease or quadriceps tie-down. These names should be considered obsolete because the problem is not always associated with a fracture and does not always involve a bridge between the femur and the quadriceps. Quadriceps contracture can develop in the absence of a femoral fracture

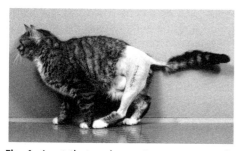
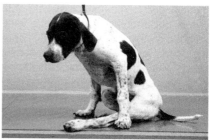

Fig. 4. A cat that underwent surgery to repair a femoral fracture is seen 14 days after surgery (*left*). The operated limb is held in excessive extension and stifle flexion is no longer possible because of a quadriceps contracture that developed during the fortnight between surgery and the reevaluation. A male pointer is presented with a quadriceps contracture (*right*). This dog had been raised with other hunting dogs and sustained no known trauma.

as a consequence of stifle joint immobilization or limb disuse. In one experimental study in dogs, pelvic limb immobilization for a 2-week period led to loss of stifle flexion but, surprisingly, less so after trauma to the quadriceps and splinting than after splinting alone, suggesting that joint immobilization is a key component of loss of stifle flexion in dogs.[22] With quadriceps contracture, the quadriceps muscle becomes fibrotic and loses all contractility. On palpation, the muscle feels as hard as bone and stifle flexion is absent. The loss of stifle motion resulting from quadriceps contracture greatly interferes with limb use. Also, the hip joint can become painful and may ultimately luxate as a result of the contracture of the rectus femoris, which is the only part of the quadriceps that originates on the pelvis.[23] The loss of ability to flex the stifle also occurs in dogs with *Neospora caninum* or *Toxoplasma gondii* infestation and can be idiopathic. A loss of ability to flex the stifles has been reported in German shepherd dogs.[24] These dogs lack the ability to flex their stifles but their quadriceps do not lose contractility. The cause of this condition is not known and efforts to help them maintain or regain stifle flexion have been unsuccessful. These dogs can have appropriate function once their cores are strengthened and once they learn to gallop (**Fig. 5**).

Loss of joint motion may also be the consequence of abnormal growth. For example, dogs with severe (grade 4) patellar luxations may have such medial displacement of the patella (and quadriceps femoris) that the quadriceps is no longer

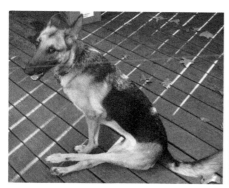
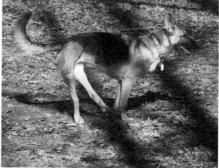

Fig. 5. A German shepherd dog lacks stifle flexion and keeps both pelvic limbs in a hyperextended position when sitting (*left*). With time, the dog can be taught to walk and run despite the lack of stifle flexion (*right*).

functioning like an extensor muscle of the stifle joint. As a consequence, the quadriceps is not stretched during stifle joint flexion and the stifle cannot be effectively extended. Within a few months, 50° or 60° of extension may be lost (**Fig. 6**). Goniometry, performed under sedation, is necessary to assess joint motion in the pelvic limbs of dogs with patellar luxation. Despite being non–weight bearing on the affected limb, some dogs with patellar luxation do not experience loss of stifle joint motion. A transient or permanent loss of carpal extension has been seen in growing dogs, particularly large-breed hunting dogs. That lack of carpal extension could be secondary to bone growth that is faster than the increase in length of the antebrachial flexor muscles (**Fig. 7**).

Loss of joint motion may be linked to neuromuscular disease or to generalized or focal myopathies. Neuromuscular diseases are often associated with abnormal muscle function, including weakness or myalgia.[25] Canine myopathies may be inflammatory, necrotizing, dystrophic, metabolic, or congenital myopathies, and a full description is beyond the scope of this article.[25–27] A dog with generalized myoclonus resulting from distemper was successfully managed by injecting botulinum toxins in the most affected muscles.[28] Focal myopathies in dogs are sometimes reported.[29] Classic syndromes include the gracilis or semitendinosus myopathy[30] often seen in German shepherd dogs and the fibrotic myopathy of the infraspinatus,[10,31–34] often seen in hunting dogs. Isolated canine myopathies have been sporadically reported in other muscles, including the supraspinatus,[10] teres major,[35] brachialis (1 cat), sartorius,[36] and iliopsoas.[37] Muscles that cross 2 joints are reportedly more prone to contractures than muscles that cross a single joint.

Excessive motion may be present in joints as a result of joint laxity or loss of muscle tone, or as a consequence of the presence of an abnormal posture or weight distribution. Joint laxity is seen is growing dogs of (large) breeds that have loose connective tissue (eg, German shepherd dogs). It often affects the areas of increased tension, particularly the palmar fibrocartilage, gastrocnemius muscle tendon complex, and to a lesser extent plantar fibrocartilage. Affected dogs may be partially or fully palmigrade or plantigrade. Carpal laxity tends to improve over time. Joint laxity is also seen

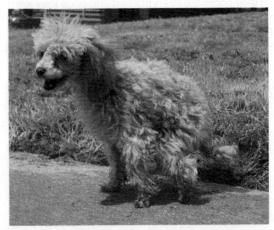

Fig. 6. An 11-month-old toy poodle has bilateral grade 4 patellar luxation. The dog has a crouched stance. Stifle joint extension is limited to ~110° rather than the anticipated ~160°. Also, the pain response to stifle joint extension is severe. This dog would ideally have had a surgical correction of his patellar luxations earlier in life, before the loss of stifle joint extension.

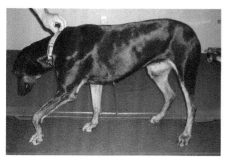 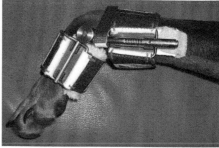

Fig. 7. A 7-month-old Doberman pinscher lacks carpal extension (*left*). Like the cat in **Fig. 1**, the presence of radial nerve palsy was suspected but an electromyogram indicated that the radial nerve and other nerves were normal. The dog was treated using a dynamic hinged brace (Pediatric Knee Extension brace system; *right*).

when growing dogs carry excessive weight on parts of their bodies. For example, fore-limb amputees that lose a leg while growing often have excessive motion of the scapula in relation to the body wall and excessive shoulder joint rotation. Also, growing dogs (of large and giant breeds) that shift weight toward their forelimbs, most often because of hip dysplasia, may develop excessive extension of the tarsus. Once the excessive extension develops, it may be permanent. Loss of muscle tone may be present in skeletally immature dogs because of disuse or immobilization. It may or may not be associated with muscle atrophy. Puppies most often develop a loss of muscle tone because of joint immobilization or because of the lack of limb use resulting from a chronically painful situation.

CLINICAL APPLICATIONS OF RANGE OF MOTION AND STRETCHING

Postoperative passive ROM should be considered in all patients but is particularly important in patients or situations in which loss of motion is anticipated, including skeletally immature dogs, after severe tissue trauma, in patients without active limb use, after trauma to the elbow or tarsus (**Fig. 8**), and after femoral fracture in cats and skeletally immature dogs. For these patients or situations, joint motion should be clearly documented and reevaluated often: daily if the problem progresses rapidly or weekly. Passive ROM and stretching must occur daily and can be delivered with the patient hospitalized or seen as an outpatient. Owner involvement should be maximized but owners should not bear the responsibility for something they may not be willing or able to do.

Stretching programs are necessary for patients that lack functionally important joint motion and should be implemented as soon as the lack of joint motion is identified because limb disuse and periarticular fibrosis tend to be self-sustaining. Stretching programs are more effective in the subacute period (1–3 weeks after injury or surgery) compared with the chronic period (>3 weeks after injury or surgery). A program can start once the acute inflammatory phase subsides; a week or so after injury or surgery. Stretching is most often done without sedation but, in rare situations, sedation may be necessary to stretch a patient.

The most critical stretching programs are done to avoid quadriceps contractures. They are implemented immediately after surgery in high-risk patients. Inpatient or daily outpatient programs are strongly recommended because owners may not recognize the signs of quadriceps contracture. Stretching after the repair of a distal femoral

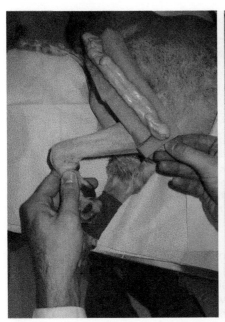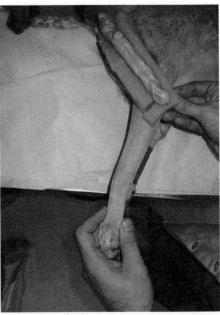

Fig. 8. A humeral fracture in a beagle has been stabilized with an external skeletal fixator with a connecting rod made of epoxy putty. Sponges were placed underneath the epoxy putty to minimize swelling and keep the skin-pin interfaces clean. Passive ROM is performed by flexing and extending the joint repeatedly with gentle pressure.

fracture in a skeletally immature dog requires little force but should take place multiple times each day. Quadriceps stretching was done successfully using a static flexion apparatus in one report involving a dog with early quadriceps contracture.[38] The stretching program subsides once stifle flexion has reached a threshold. Subjectively, once the stifle can flex to ∼60° and once the patient is actively flexing the stifle and bearing weight on the limb, quadriceps contracture becomes unlikely.

The most common clinical situation that warrants a stretching program is a dog presenting with pelvic limb disuse as a result of a femoral head ostectomy. In these dogs, limb disuse is most often caused by the combination of severe pain during hip extension and the lack of hip extension (**Fig. 9**). Increasing hip extension is key to managing these patients. Once extension increases, the residual pain that is perceived in full extension is outside the hip ROM used at a walk and trot, and the dog can strengthen the limb through exercise. Dogs also commonly present with lack of stifle extension after extracapsular stabilization or TPLO.[39] After extracapsular stabilization, the loss of extension may be related to the location of the tibial tunnel for the stabilizing suture loop. Restriction of extension is likely if the tibial tunnel is too distal. After TPLO, a loss of extension greater than 10° is uncommon (<3% in one study) but it is associated with increased lameness and decreased response to physical rehabilitation.[39] General physical rehabilitation increases stifle flexion and extension after TPLO.[40] For patients that lack joint motion 3 weeks after surgery, a stretching program that involves heating and stretching should be considered. A stretching program should similarly be considered any time an injured patient presents with a loss of motion after surgery, particularly after any fracture repair but also with any fracture involving an open growth plate (because the patient is young and growing), involving the elbow or tarsus (because these joints seem to be most vulnerable to loss of motion), or associated with severe

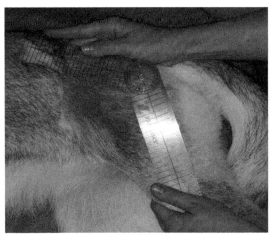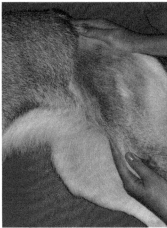

Fig. 9. A 1-year-old Siberian husky has left pelvic limb disuse after a femoral head ostectomy performed 2 months earlier. A severe pain response to hip extension combined with a 35° lack of hip extension is present at the time of initial evaluation (*left*). Therapy included heating the hip region with a moist heat pack, stretching the hip primary to gain extension (*right*), and the design of an exercise program that included limb use.

tissue trauma or infection (because more tissue trauma or infection yields more fibrosis). Patients undergoing limb lengthening often need stretching of the joint distal to the bone being lengthened. It is often possible to connect bars to the distal aspect of a circular external fixator and connect a sling made of self-adhesive bandage material to these bars to achieve safe and convenient low-torque sustained stretching.[41]

Loss of range motion is a key feature of OA. In humans, features of articular degeneration are associated with reduced knee ROM and reduced hip ROM in patients with early OA. Pain, stiffness, higher body mass index, and male gender are associated with reduced ROM as well.[42] Stretching is beneficial to some dogs and cats with chronic OA. As mentioned earlier, not all patients with OA lose joint motion and few lose enough joint motion to have clinical consequences. In a study evaluating Labrador retrievers with hip dysplasia, loss of extension was associated with an increase in clinical signs.[18] Also, a more active lifestyle was associated with less lameness in these dogs. Because exercise stretches and increases strength, it is logical to keep dogs with OA as active as tolerated. Subjectively, it seems that tighter joints with OA lose more motion than looser joints with OA. For example, large losses of elbow and tarsal flexion are common with OA. It is not known whether staying active could decrease these losses. In patients with significant loss of joint motion, stretching through exercise should be considered first. Land-based exercise and aquatic exercises are equally beneficial to ROM in humans with knee OA.[43] Manual stretching should be considered for patients with OA with severe loss of joint motion that cannot exercise. Progress is likely to be slow because of chronicity and ideally the owner should get involved to reduce the cost of care. A small pilot study in 10 dogs with OA suggested that home-based stretching programs are beneficial to patients with OA.[44] Patients with OA can also see gains in joint ROM. Increased hip flexion was present in dogs with OA in one study and an increase in ROM in the shoulder, elbow, carpus, and tarsus, was present in cats with OA in another.[18,45] Increases in joint motion are likely caused by loss of muscle mass for joint positions with soft tissue approximation end feels (see **Table 1**). Patients recovering from total joint arthroplasty may need a stretching program, because most joint replacements are done in joints with severe OA that are likely to lack joint motion. In dogs, loss of joint motion seems more likely after total knee and elbow replacement, compared with hip replacement. With a stretching program that involves manual stretching replaced over time by controlled exercises, significant gains in joint motion can be achieved.[46]

Stretching for joint health is done often in performance dogs, including dogs that race, track, perform agility, work, and do conformation. As mentioned earlier, little is known about optimal stretching parameters and the impact of stretching on injury rate and performance. It is therefore logical to follow a general approach to warm-up and cool-down exercises without being dogmatic about specific parameters. Warming up can include walking for a few minutes followed by gentle manual stretching of forelimbs and hind limbs. Stretching should be performed immediately before exercise because the effects of stretching on joint motion are short lived, lasting only 6 minutes in one study.[47] Warming up does not make muscles less stiff or longer; it only influences stretch tolerance.[48]

REFERENCES

1. Jaegger G, Marcellin-Little DJ, Levine D. Reliability of goniometry in Labrador Retrievers. Am J Vet Res 2002;63:979–86.
2. Jaeger GH, Marcellin-Little DJ, Depuy V, et al. Validity of goniometric joint measurements in cats. Am J Vet Res 2007;68:822–6.
3. Thomas TM, Marcellin-Little DJ, Roe SC, et al. Comparison of measurements obtained by use of an electrogoniometer and a universal plastic goniometer for the assessment of joint motion in dogs. Am J Vet Res 2006;67:1974–9.
4. Agostinho FS, Rahal SC, Miqueleto NS, et al. Kinematic analysis of Labrador Retrievers and Rottweilers trotting on a treadmill. Vet Comp Orthop Traumatol 2011; 24:185–91.
5. Brady RB, Sidiropoulos AN, Bennett HJ, et al. Evaluation of gait-related variables in lean and obese dogs at a trot. Am J Vet Res 2013;74:757–62.
6. Marcellin-Little DJ, Ferretti A, Roe SC, et al. Hinged Ilizarov external fixation for correction of antebrachial deformities. Vet Surg 1998;27:231–45.
7. Feeney LC, Lin CF, Marcellin-Little DJ, et al. Validation of two-dimensional kinematic analysis of walk and sit-to-stand motions in dogs. Am J Vet Res 2007;68: 277–82.
8. Cook JL, Renfro DC, Tomlinson JL, et al. Measurement of angles of abduction for diagnosis of shoulder instability in dogs using goniometry and digital image analysis. Vet Surg 2005;34:463–8.
9. van Bree H. Vacuum phenomenon associated with osteochondrosis of the scapulohumeral joint in dogs: 100 cases (1985-1991). J Am Vet Med Assoc 1992;201: 1916–7.
10. Marcellin-Little DJ, Levine D, Canapp SO Jr. The canine shoulder: selected disorders and their management with physical therapy. Clin Tech Small Anim Pract 2007;22:171–82.
11. Piper TL, Whiteside LA. Early mobilization after knee ligament repair in dogs: an experimental study. Clin Orthop Relat Res 1980;(150):277–82.
12. Levine D, Millis DL, Marcellin-Little DJ. Introduction to veterinary physical rehabilitation. Vet Clin North Am Small Anim Pract 2005;35:1247–54, vii.
13. Levine D, Marcellin-Little DJ, Millis DL, et al. Effects of partial immersion in water on vertical ground reaction forces and weight distribution in dogs. Am J Vet Res 2010;71:1413–6.

14. Herbert RD, Gabriel M. Effects of stretching before and after exercising on muscle soreness and risk of injury: systematic review. BMJ 2002;325:468.
15. Nicholson HL, Osmotherly PG, Smith BA, et al. Determinants of passive hip range of motion in adult Greyhounds. Aust Vet J 2007;85:217–21.
16. Usuba M, Akai M, Shirasaki Y, et al. Experimental joint contracture correction with low torque–long duration repeated stretching. Clin Orthop Relat Res 2007;(456): 70–8.
17. Usuba M, Miyanaga Y, Miyakawa S, et al. Effect of heat in increasing the range of knee motion after the development of a joint contracture: an experiment with an animal model. Arch Phys Med Rehabil 2006;87:247–53.
18. Greene LM, Marcellin-Little DJ, Lascelles BD. Associations among exercise duration, lameness severity, and hip joint range of motion in Labrador Retrievers with hip dysplasia. J Am Vet Med Assoc 2013;242:1528–33.
19. Moeller EM, Allen DA, Wilson ER, et al. Long-term outcomes of thigh circumference, stifle range-of-motion, and lameness after unilateral tibial plateau levelling osteotomy. Vet Comp Orthop Traumatol 2010;23:37–42.
20. Millis DL. Responses of musculoskeletal tissues to disuse and remobilization. In: Millis DL, Levine D, editors. Canine rehabilitation and physical therapy. 2nd edition. Philadelphia: Saunders; 2014. p. 92–153.
21. Fries CL, Binnington AG, Cockshutt JR. Quadriceps contracture in four cats: a complication of internal fixation of femoral fractures. Vet Comp Orthop Traumatol 1988;2:91–6.
22. Shires PK, Braund KG, Milton JL, et al. Effect of localized trauma and temporary splinting on immature skeletal muscle and mobility of the femorotibial joint in the dog. Am J Vet Res 1982;43:454–60.
23. Bardet JF, Hohn RB. Quadriceps contracture in dogs. J Am Vet Med Assoc 1983; 183:680–5.
24. Straight leg shepherds. Available at: www.straightlegshepherds.org. Accessed August 14, 2014.
25. Shelton GD. Routine and specialized laboratory testing for the diagnosis of neuromuscular diseases in dogs and cats. Vet Clin Pathol 2010;39:278–95.
26. Shelton GD. From dog to man: the broad spectrum of inflammatory myopathies. Neuromuscul Disord 2007;17:663–70.
27. Evans J, Levesque D, Shelton GD. Canine inflammatory myopathies: a clinico-pathologic review of 200 cases. J Vet Intern Med 2004;18:679–91.
28. Schubert T, Clemmons R, Miles S, et al. The use of botulinum toxin for the treatment of generalized myoclonus in a dog. J Am Anim Hosp Assoc 2013;49:122–7.
29. Taylor J, Tangner CH. Acquired muscle contractures in the dog and cat. A review of the literature and case report. Vet Comp Orthop Traumatol 2007;20:79–85.
30. Lewis DD, Shelton GD, Piras A, et al. Gracilis or semitendinosus myopathy in 18 dogs. J Am Anim Hosp Assoc 1997;33:177–88.
31. Dillon EA, Anderson LJ, Jones BR. Infraspinatus muscle contracture in a working dog. N Z Vet J 1989;37:32–4.
32. Harasen G. Infraspinatus muscle contracture. Can Vet J 2005;46:751–2.
33. Pettit GD. Infraspinatus muscle contracture in dogs. Mod Vet Pract 1980;61: 451–2.
34. Devor M, Sorby R. Fibrotic contracture of the canine infraspinatus muscle: pathophysiology and prevention by early surgical intervention. Vet Comp Orthop Traumatol 2006;19:117–21.
35. Bruce WJ, Spence S, Miller A. Teres minor myopathy as a cause of lameness in a dog. J Small Anim Pract 1997;38:74–7.

36. Lobetti RG, Hill TP. Sartorius muscle contracture in a dog. J S Afr Vet Assoc 1994; 65:28–30.

37. Adrega Da Silva C, Bernard F, Bardet JF, et al. Fibrotic myopathy of the iliopsoas muscle in a dog. Vet Comp Orthop Traumatol 2009;22:238–42.

38. Moores AP, Sutton A. Management of quadriceps contracture in a dog using a static flexion apparatus and physiotherapy. J Small Anim Pract 2009;50:251–4.

39. Jandi AS, Schulman AJ. Incidence of motion loss of the stifle joint in dogs with naturally occurring cranial cruciate ligament rupture surgically treated with tibial plateau leveling osteotomy: longitudinal clinical study of 412 cases. Vet Surg 2007;36:114–21.

40. Monk ML, Preston CA, McGowan CM. Effects of early intensive postoperative physiotherapy on limb function after tibial plateau leveling osteotomy in dogs with deficiency of the cranial cruciate ligament. J Am Vet Med Assoc 2006; 228:725.

41. Kwan TW, Marcellin-Little DJ, Harrysson OL. Correction of biapical radial deformities by use of bi-level hinged circular external fixation and distraction osteogenesis in 13 dogs. Vet Surg 2014;43:316–29.

42. Holla JF, Steultjens MP, van der Leeden M, et al. Determinants of range of joint motion in patients with early symptomatic osteoarthritis of the hip and/or knee: an exploratory study in the CHECK cohort. Osteoarthritis Cartilage 2011;19: 411–9.

43. Wyatt FB, Milam S, Manske RC, et al. The effects of aquatic and traditional exercise programs on persons with knee osteoarthritis. J Strength Cond Res 2001;15: 337–40.

44. Crook T, McGowan C, Pead M. Effect of passive stretching on the range of motion of osteoarthritic joints in 10 Labrador Retrievers. Vet Rec 2007;160:545–7.

45. Lascelles BD, Dong YH, Marcellin-Little DJ, et al. Relationship of orthopedic examination, goniometric measurements, and radiographic signs of degenerative joint disease in cats. BMC Vet Res 2012;8:10.

46. Liska WD, Marcellin-Little DJ, Eskelinen EV, et al. Custom total knee replacement in a dog with femoral condylar bone loss. Vet Surg 2007;36:293–301.

47. Spernoga SG, Uhl TL, Arnold BL, et al. Duration of maintained hamstring flexibility after a one-time, modified hold-relax stretching protocol. J Athl Train 2001;36: 44–8.

48. Halbertsma JP, Goeken LN. Stretching exercises: effect on passive extensibility and stiffness in short hamstrings of healthy subjects. Arch Phys Med Rehabil 1994;75:976–81.

Principles and Applications of Therapeutic Exercises for Small Animals

Marti G. Drum, DVM, PhD[a], Denis J. Marcellin-Little, DEDV[b],*,
Michael S. Davis, DVM, PhD[c]

KEYWORDS

- Therapeutic exercise • Underwater treadmill • Strengthening • Proprioception
- Balance • Endurance

KEY POINTS

- Therapeutic exercises to increase active ROM, strength, endurance, speed, and proprioception are the cornerstone of rehabilitation and conditioning programs.
- Therapeutic exercise programs used for rehabilitation are designed to bring injured and dysfunctional limbs back to a level comparable with uninjured limbs, beginning with low-level activities and progressing to higher-level activities.
- Therapeutic exercise programs should be designed so that all involved tissues are challenged for strengthening, but not so rapidly as to result in complications and tissue damage.
- Variety is essential to prevent the owner and patient from becoming bored and allowing appropriate progression of load and tissues.
- Exercise programs used for conditioning increase strength and fitness of all limbs. They are tailored to the activities the patient is expected to perform.

Therapeutic exercise is a cornerstone of rehabilitation and is used to improve active joint range of motion (ROM), improve weight bearing and limb use, build strength and muscle mass, and increase conditioning (endurance, speed, and so forth). Each case is unique as chronicity, type of injury, patient signalment and temperament, owner compliance, and level of required functional recovery. For example, a military or police working German Shepherd dog must return to a much higher performance level than a family companion German Shepherd dog. Additionally, therapeutic

[a] Department of Small Animal Clinical Sciences, College of Veterinary Medicine, University of Tennessee, 2407 River Drive, Knoxville, TN 37996, USA; [b] Department of Clinical Sciences, College of Veterinary Medicine, North Carolina State University, NCSU CVM VHC #2563, 1052 William Moore Drive, Raleigh, NC 27607–4065, USA; [c] Department of Physiological Sciences, Center for Veterinary Health Sciences, Oklahoma State University, 264 McElroy Hall, Stillwater, OK 74078, USA
* Corresponding author. NCSU CVM VHC #2563, 1052 William Moore Drive, Raleigh, NC 27607.
E-mail address: djmarcel@ncsu.edu

Vet Clin Small Anim 45 (2015) 73–90
http://dx.doi.org/10.1016/j.cvsm.2014.09.005
0195-5616/15/$ – see front matter © 2015 Elsevier Inc. All rights reserved.

exercise is essential for partial return to working or performance. For example, a performance agility dog may be able to return to competition, but at a lower level that requires lower jump heights, fewer obstacles, and so forth.

TYPES OF EXERCISE

Broadly, exercises are either closed kinetic chain or open kinetic chain exercises. Closed chain exercises are typically weight-bearing exercises that require multiple muscle groups to contract simultaneously while the limbs remain in contact with the ground. Open chain exercises are targeted exercises where the paw has a period of non–weight-bearing activity, such as the "shake hands" exercise for elbow flexion and shoulder extension. Closed chain exercises, such as jumping or rising, are thought to have better functional benefits than open chain exercises.[1] Closed chain exercises can also be combined with proprioceptive exercises, such as performing activities on a Physioroll (FitBALL Peanut, Ball Dynamics International, Longmont, CO, USA) (standing, sit-to-stands, lateral bending, and so forth) and thus further increasing neuromuscular re-education and core muscle activation. Another way to classify exercises is based on their purpose, such as exercises aimed at promoting joint motion, proprioceptive, strength and endurance, core stability, and speed exercises. Many exercises are combination exercises because they accomplish multiple goals simultaneously.

Although strength and endurance conditioning are important to any exercise regime, exercise programs should focus on functional goals. For example, endurance is key to hunting and tracking dogs, whereas strength and explosiveness is key to racing and lure coursing. Strength exercises are performed with maximal or near-maximal muscle contraction, with relatively few repetitions, which results in muscle hypertrophy over time. In contrast, endurance exercises are those that are performed with repetitive contractions over a prolonged time, with relatively little load applied to the muscle. In contrast to strength training aerobic capacity, but not muscle fiber diameter, increases with endurance activities. Although most weight loss results from dietary adjustments, exercise, and particularly low-intensity, long-duration exercise should be a key component of weight loss programs to prevent lean muscle mass loss from caloric restriction.

Core stability involves the abdominal wall, pelvic floor, diaphragm, and lower back. The importance of strong core body muscles is emphasized in human rehabilitation and training, and has become popular in canine sports training. Strong core muscles make it easier to perform many physical activities, but it still remains to be proved that core strengthening programs prevent injury.

Speed exercises are important in the final phases of an exercise protocol, and these phases must not occur before adequate tissue healing, muscle strength, and endurance have occurred to prevent possible injury or reinjury. Trotting, running, and running on a treadmill are all methods to increase speed in dogs. Interval training is a noncontinuous form of activity that includes brief rest periods between repeated exercises. Intervals are very useful in speed training where near-maximal effort is used, followed by a less intense effort. Repetitions of high/low intensity exercises are then repeated and increased as tolerated. Another strategy is a pyramid or "build up/build down" approach, particularly in designing treadmill-based programs.

Plyometrics, or explosive jump training, requires various jumps in place without taking a stride to generate serial jumping. Simply, plyometrics cause a rapid stretch of the muscle followed immediately by the shortening of a muscle group during dynamic activity.[2] Plyometrics greatly increase the force on the muscle, facilitating increased strength and power. This occurs by attaining a higher active muscle state before short-ening and potentiating muscle activation via the stretch reflex.[2] Thus, plyometrics are commonly thought to increase power and speed. Caution should be exercised when prescribing plyometrics because drop jumping generates loads of up to 10 times body mass in humans. The increase in loads generated during jumps in dogs is not known. Unfortunately, plyometrics can be difficult to design for most dogs, but often the patients that benefit from plyometrics are highly trained and are therefore easier to train (**Fig. 1**).

Examples of activities commonly used in therapeutic exercise programs include weight shifting and balance work, targeted core strengthening exercises, stair climb-ing, sit-to-stand exercises, treadmill activity with resistance or incline work, "dancing" (for rear limb activity), Cavaletti rails (Medium Cavaletti, Affordable Agility, Bloomfield, NY, USA), controlled ball and toy play (fetch or tug), underwater treadmill (UWTM) ex-ercises, and swimming. This is an abbreviated list because specific exercises are only limited by the therapist's imagination. More than 400 therapeutic exercises are used in human physical therapy. When designing an exercise protocol for a patient, the most important factor is to identify the patient's problems and limitations. These limitations may be the consequence of the surgical procedure, of a particular muscle group pain or weakness, of joint restrictions, of the fitness level of the patient, and often most significantly of the patient's motivation level. Routine re-evaluation of the patient is recommended to assess the adaptations that are occurring during rehabilitation and to determine the appropriate rate of progression. Additionally, home exercises should be regularly monitored to ensure proper form and technique are being followed by the client.

SPECIAL CONSIDERATIONS DURING EXERCISE

Good footing to avoid slipping is paramount to any exercise regimen, particularly for weak patients or during high-intensity activities. It is important to have adequate space to perform exercises with as little distraction as possible especially in the clinic, where other dogs can be distracting to patients.

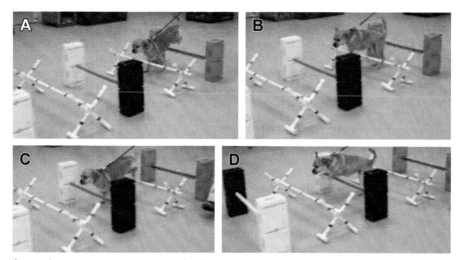

Fig. 1. Plyometric exercise using multiple jumps to create a bounce activity. Images *A–D* are in series, as the patient performs the activity.

Recognition of fatigue is another essential element of designing exercise programs. Refusal to do a particular task, performing a task poorly, vocalizing (whining, barking, or even growling or snapping), limb trembling, and increased lameness are some signs of fatigue and/or pain that would signal the end of a specific exercise set. However, a brief rest lasting 2 to 3 minutes may be all that is needed in active patients. Fatigue can be caused by either insufficient energy or hyperthermia, so particular attention should be directed to respiratory rate in high-intensity activities, such as swimming or jogging on the treadmill in which the rate of metabolic heat generation can exceed the ability of the dog to dissipate that heat. In addition, athletic dogs that have experienced substantial loss of fitness because of prolonged inactivity or obese patients may be particularly impaired in metabolic heat dissipation and hyperventilation often is the earliest indicator of fatigue.

Exercise sessions should always be positive, which can be challenging when introducing higher-level tasks or in patients that are apprehensive. Patients that are food or toy motivated are obviously easier to train, but even food-motivated dogs can be difficult to motivate when faced with a new and unusual object, activity, or scenario. Often, release of pressure from the leash or from gentle manual touch in combination with verbal praise immediately when the movement, behavior, or task is initiated can be the most powerful method of training. Clicker training, which is a training method that uses positive reinforcement and an audible click to mark the desired behavior, can be useful in teaching complex behaviors and activities.[3] As a general rule, modifications to home exercise programs should be made once or twice weekly, and changes to outpatient therapy should be made every one to three sessions, depending on patient tolerance.

PRACTICAL EXERCISES

The following is a practical guide to some common exercises used in therapeutic exercise protocols. A more exhaustive list and description of exercises used in dogs is available in the literature.[3]

Land Treadmill

Land treadmills are excellent tools for a variety of exercises ranging from improving limb use after surgery to increasing strength and endurance in high-level athletes. Dogs that are trained to walk on leash generally are easily trained to walk on a treadmill. Patients should always be directly supervised and closely monitored for signs of fatigue, such as pulling on the harness, stumbling, or drifting side to side. Human treadmills can be used, but are at a disadvantage compared with canine-specific treadmills because canine treadmills generally have longer belts that enable medium and large dogs to trot safely and comfortably, begin at a lower speed (0.2 m/s [0.5 mph] or less), and have railing or gates on the sides to discourage jumping off the treadmill. Nonelectric treadmills are not recommended for dogs, because it is difficult for most dogs to initiate the treadmill belt movement. Treadmill placement is also important. Treadmills should be placed such that the dog is not facing a wall or in a manner such that frequent distractions are behind the dog. It is also important that a handler is able to be in front of and beside the dog, particularly during treadmill training. Positive rewards in the form of food, vocal praise, or toys are essential, but are only part of the training process. Release of pressure in the form of stopping the treadmill belt as soon as the dog voluntarily walks forward is just as important as food, verbal, or toy encouragement. Several repetitions of short (2- to 10-second long) intervals are more successful and often less stressful than one prolonged episode during treadmill introduction. Once the dog begins to understand he or she is expected to walk forward on the treadmill, increasing durations of walking can be performed. Some dogs may only need one or two short training periods before they are comfortably walking several minutes continuously. However, many dogs hesitate or challenge the treadmill walking by stepping off the sides, riding the belt back, or attempting to jump off the front of the treadmill even after several successful minutes of comfortable walking. Thus, it is important that two handlers are available during training so that one can be encouraging in front and preventing the dog from jumping forward. The second handler can direct leash control to prevent stepping on the nonmoving sides or riding too far toward the back or front of the treadmill. It is also recommended to begin with a harness for training for more comfortable control of the dog's body mass and to prevent excessive pulling on the neck. In some cases, both a leash and a harness can be used for maximum control. Canine treadmills with sides can be configured such that bungee cords, or other straps, connect to the harness to help keep the dog in the center of the treadmill.

Exercise considerations
A warm-up period of walking and then fast walking is recommended before trotting on a treadmill. It is important that the treadmill speed be rapidly increased when changing gait from a walk to a trot to avoid an awkward transition. In general, most medium to large dogs walk comfortably at a rate of 0.9 to 1.2 m/s (2–2.7 mph). A medium trot is generally 1.7 to 2 m/s (3.8–4.5 mph). Walking or jogging duration and speed can be increased to advance endurance, but the treadmill may also be angled up or down to reduce or increase the forces placed on the forelimbs or rear limbs for specific strengthening of the target limb or limbs. Interval training and gait transition exercises are easy to accomplish with a land treadmill. Many dogs recovering from orthopedic or neurologic injuries have significant difficulties with transitioning from the walk to trot and vice versa, whereas athletic and power building exercises are best accomplished by interval programs that vary the speed and incline. Lateral work can be accomplished by using a solid block or human exercise step, and placing the forelimbs on the treadmill and hind limbs on the solid object or vice versa. This is a very high level exercise for many dogs, and should only be attempted once they are comfortable with regular treadmill exercise. Similarly, targeted forelimb and hind limb work can be done by placing the solid block or step at the end of the treadmill such that only the forelimbs or hind limbs are moving, while the opposite pair of limbs is stationary. For these advanced exercises, a harness is essential to support the patient during the training process, and the treadmill should be started at a very slow speed. Further challenges can be introduced by replacing the solid object with an unstable surface, such as a Physioroll. Thus, these advanced treadmill exercises not only can be beneficial for isolated limb strengthening, but also for core activation and strengthening. Additional modifications, such as resistance bands and leg weights during treadmill exercise, are discussed later.

Core Strengthening

Many exercises focus on core strength. These exercises include sit-to-stands or down-to-stands on ball, Physioroll, or trampoline; walking with a rolling object; rolling over; rolling slowly to pause in each direction; sit-ups and crunches with or without holds or twists; two-legged standing; begging; praying; bowing; and four-direction stretches on a Physioroll (**Fig. 2**). Caution should be used in performing any of these exercises in dogs with back, hip, or shoulder problems. In general, core-strength exercises may be repeated five times. As core strength increases, they can be increased

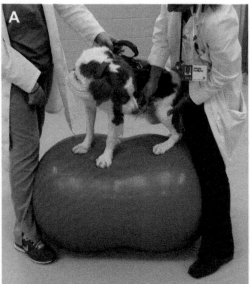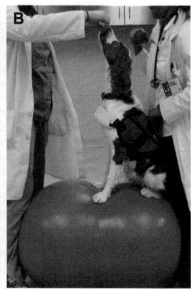

Fig. 2. Core strengthening exercises using a physioroll. (*A*) Directional "cookie" stretches on the physioroll work on flexibility while activating core musculature. (*B*) Sitting on the physioroll with a reach for spinal extension as part of advanced sit-to-stand exercises.

to 10 to 15 repetitions, two to three times daily. A combination of exercises allows strengthening of different muscle groups, while preventing boredom.

Rhythmic Stabilization

Rhythmic stabilization is a technique used to strengthen postural muscles in dogs. In particular; this exercise is valuable for strengthening the triceps and quadriceps muscle groups. It also helps to provide neuromuscular feedback to joints, ligaments, and muscle-tendon units. Rhythmic stabilization should be performed on an unstable surface, such as a therapy ball or roll, trampoline, or inflated mattress. With the animal standing squarely, the therapist places gentle pressure over the pelvis or cranial thoracic region and gently "bounces" the animal up and down (**Fig. 3**). The bouncing motion should be relatively rapid, with only enough recovery time to regain the normal standing position. This generates rapid firing of postural muscles in an isometric fashion, which is ideal for weakly ambulatory or significantly ataxic patients.

Cavaletti Rails

The primary result of Cavaletti rail walking is an increase in elbow, stifle, and hock flexion and gait alterations (ie, stride lengthening). They may also be used to challenge proprioception, balance, and coordination in animals returning to function following neurologic impairment. Varying the widths and heights of the rails can further challenge the patient and change how the core musculature is used. Unstable surfaces (foam) or balance equipment (discs or Fit Bones [Ball Dynamics, International, Longmont, CO, USA]) increase the difficulty level for most all patients (**Fig. 4**).

Exercise design

Cavaletti rails may be commercially purchased or can be created by the savvy therapist or client. Two or more poles may be used and should be spaced at appropriate distances apart, determined by the dog's natural stride length (**Fig. 5**). Four to ten rails

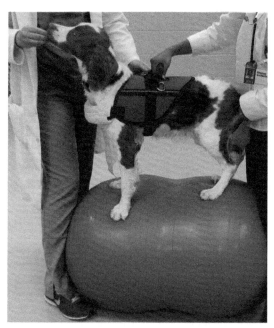

Fig. 3. Rhythmic stabilization on a physioroll. Often two people are needed for this exercise, one to keep the patient's attention and stabilize the ball, the other to rhythmically bounce the patient while maintaining a standing position. A harness is helpful for this exercise.

are preferable, particularly if stride lengthening is a primary goal. The distance between rails is ideally just wide enough to allow for a single step between the rails at a normal gait speed. The faster the gait, the wider the poles should be placed. To begin, poles should be just slightly above the dog's carpus. In very short dogs, such as Dachshunds, the rails may be taped to the ground if standard heights are too tall. Also, significantly paretic animals may need very low poles to begin to actually step over the rails instead of dragging the affected limbs over each rail. Patience is key because the first step over a rail can be very intimidating to some dogs. Begin with walking 5 to 10 times over the rails, and progress to 10 to 20 times over the rails. The more numerous the Cavaletti rails, the fewer repetitions are needed. Progress from a walk to trot with uniform Cavaletti rails. If a patient is unable or is restricted from trotting, alternating heights, adding an unstable surface, varying the widths

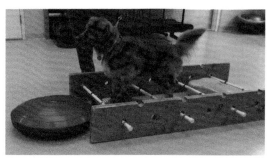

Fig. 4. Cavaletti rails with increased difficulty by adding balance disk and FitBones to standard Cavaletti rails.

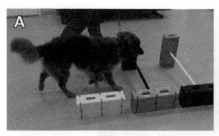 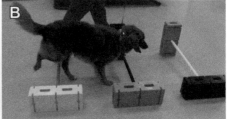

Fig. 5. Basic Cavaletti rails. Note the increased elbow flexion (*A*) and stifle flexion (*B*) during this activity.

and number of poles (**Fig. 6**), or incorporating into a circle are ways to advance the exercise.

Incline Exercise

Pelvic limb ROM increases when walking up an incline: climbing up an inclined surface promotes increased flexion, extension, and ROM of the hip.[4] However, stifle flexion is decreased. Walking up an inclined ramp also results in greater ROM of the forelimb joints. Shoulder extension and ROM, elbow flexion and extension, and carpal flexion are greater when walking up a ramp compared with ascending stairs or trotting over level ground.[4] However, patients with joint restrictions (decreased hip or shoulder extension) may alter their gait resulting in a shorter stride length. Depending on exercise goals, exercises other than using inclines may be more useful to increase the ROM of specific joints. In contrast, incline walking may improve limb use because of the shift in the patient's center of gravity. Inclines may also be useful for gait retraining or to stimulate proprioception. It is important to begin on a gentle incline for many patients. Secure footing is essential for all patients. An easy solution to reducing the slippery surface on many ramps or manufactured inclines is the use of rubber yoga mats or bath mats with rubber backing.

Exercise design

One can use either time or repetitions to define the exercise interval. For example, if using a plastic or metal ramp designed for loading into vehicles, one might begin with 5 to 10 repetitions, once to three times daily. Most dogs must be acclimated to this style of ramp, and both ends must be secure to prevent wobbling or moving during exercise. Begin with walking on the ramp flat on the ground and gradually increase the

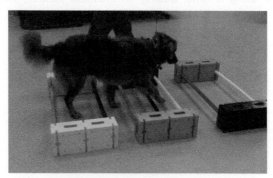

Fig. 6. Adding rails, varying gait speed, changing widths or height of rails are simple ways to challenge a patient further during Cavaletti exercise.

angle of inclination. More commonly, grassy hills are readily available to most every patient. Unfortunately, hills may be too steep for patients, especially in the early phases of recovery. An easy method to incorporate inclines into the exercise regime is to add incline walking to part of the regular leash walks the patient should be performing. A gradual incline is found and incorporated into the walking path, but repetitions should be instituted not just a single pass during the walking path. For example, a patient may need to walk 5 minutes to reach the incline, then perform 5 to 10 repetitions, then continue the remainder of the walk. If only steep inclines are available, walking up in a gentle serpentine fashion is often easier for the patient. Additionally, walking diagonally or tight serpentines, varying the speed of the inclines, adding resistance (exercise bands attached to the affected limb and pet's harness, weight vests or backpacks, dragging or pulling weight, and so forth), or limb weights are methods to advance this exercise. When advancing, begin by adding the additional challenge to 50% of the exercise and increase as tolerated.

Stair Climbing

Climbing stairs is useful to improve ROM, power in the rear limb extensors, coordination, and proprioception; in many instances, it is an activity of daily living that must be performed in the home environment. Strength building of the quadriceps and gluteal muscle groups is targeted when the limb pushes off each step. Extension of both the hips and knees is increased while propelling the body up the steps.[5] When this is difficult for patients, they may hop, trip, or refuse to do the exercise. Reducing the number of steps or the height or width of steps, or actively assisting during ascent and descent may be necessary for weak or deconditioned patients.

Climbing stairs is also beneficial for increasing ROM of the pelvic limb joints because they are significantly increased during stair climbing compared with trotting on level ground.[6] Although extension of the hip and hock joints is moderately increased with stair climbing, flexion of the stifle and hock joints seem to contribute significantly to ascending stairs by flexing these joints to raise the limb up to the height of the step. This may be particularly useful in neurologic cases where hock and stifle flexion is limited by weakness or peroneal nerve palsy. In the forelimb, shoulder extension is less and flexion is greater with stair climbing compared with trotting over ground.[7] Elbow and carpal flexion, extension, and overall ROM are greater with stair ascent as compared with trotting over ground.

Exercise design

Stairs should be introduced slowly because this is a challenging exercise for the musculoskeletal and cardiovascular systems. Fatigue may occur quickly, so it is recommended to begin with two to five sets initially. A set of steps is considered up and down 5 to 10 steps. Standard stair height (approximately 16 cm per 6 in) is appropriate for large-breed dogs but is very challenging to small patients. For small patients, half-steps or ramps are more manageable. Also, foam pieces, or blocks (Balance Pad, Ball Dynamics International, Longmont, CO, USA) can be used to decrease the stair height. Stair construction (open vs closed riders, material, traction) greatly impacts the dogs' comfort level during stair climbing and descent. In the deconditioned or ataxic patient, descent is often the most challenging part of stair exercises. Chest harnesses are useful in controlling speed when introducing stair climbing. Beyond increasing number of repetitions, "stop and go" stairs, trotting stairs, or adding weighted vests are ways to increase the challenge. In the motivated patient, walking backward up or down stairs represents an additional significant challenge.

Sit-to-Stand Exercises

Sit-to-stand exercises help strengthen hip and stifle extensor muscles and improve active ROM. The act of sitting, then standing up, requires muscle strength of the gluteal, quadriceps, hamstring, and gastrocnemius muscle groups. Sit-to-stand exercise results in greater flexion of the tarsus and nearly twice as much flexion of the stifle and hip, whereas extension of these joints is less, as compared with walking.[8]

Exercise design

Most patients already know a sit command, so little training is needed for this exercise. However, some dogs may not be taught to sit purposely, such as show dogs. It is extremely important to perform these exercises correctly because pulling a leg under the body or excessively abducting limbs shifts the force onto a single hind limb (**Fig. 7**). A brief warm up on leash is needed before beginning, and 5 to 10 repetitions twice daily are initially recommended. Although it is most beneficial if the patient sits and stands within the confined area, this is too challenging for most patients. A more successful approach is to ask for a "sit," then the handler takes one step backward and asks the patient to "come" or "stand." Once the patient is stronger and more familiar with the exercise, the handler can work toward performing the exercise in a finite area.

Sit-to-stand exercises are particularly helpful in cases of hip osteoarthritis. Hip extension is particularly painful in cases of hip osteoarthritis, and sit-to-stand allows

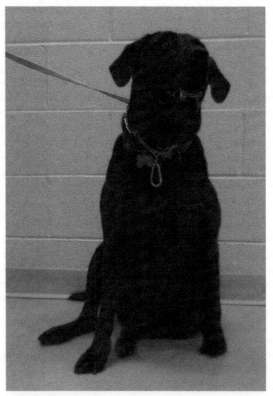

Fig. 7. An uneven sit because of partial cranial cruciate ligament tear. During sit-to-stand exercises, it is imperative that the patient sit squarely so that the affected limb is used during the exercise.

for gluteal muscle activation and active ROM without significant hip extension. Each patient must be assessed to be certain that sit-to-stands are not too stressful or painful for that individual. If normal sit-to-stands are too painful, or the patient is too weak to rise from a sitting position, several modifications may be implemented. Doing sit-to-stands with the pelvis in an elevated position may be helpful in patients that are too weak to rise from a complete sitting position. Dogs may sit with their pelvis on a stool, stair step, stack of books, curb, firm cushion, or the therapist's leg or knee and rise from this elevated position (**Fig. 8**). Many dogs need guidance from the therapist's hands to learn to sit on an object because it is a foreign concept for many patients. Alternatively, dogs may be assisted with a sling from a sitting to a standing position.

Dogs may also do sit-to-stands on an incline, with the body facing downhill to make it easier to stand. Alternatively, dogs may do sit-to-stands on an incline with the body facing uphill or sideways to each direction to provide an additional challenge and greater strengthening. For this challenge, dogs may perform five repetitions in each direction for a total of 20 repetitions, twice daily. If Physioroll, donut, or balance disks are available, challenges can be added by placing either forelimbs or hind limbs on an unstable surface (**Fig. 9**).

Tunnels and Limbo Dance

Agility training tunnels or children's play tunnels may be used to promote flexion in the forelimbs and rear limbs while strengthening the supporting muscles that hold the joints in this more flexed position. The size of the tunnel opening should be slightly shorter than the dog's standing height. The dog is encouraged to crouch low and walk through the tunnel, which requires greater limb flexion and strength than that needed for normal walking. Greater challenges may be instituted by using tunnels that are even smaller as dogs strengthen their muscles.

Because tunnels may not be available to a therapist or client, a telescoping pole, such as a shower rail, may be adjusted in a doorway, with the height slightly lower than the dorsal midline. The dog then walks under the pole to perform the exercise resembling a limbo dance (**Fig. 10**). The pole may be lowered to challenge the dog

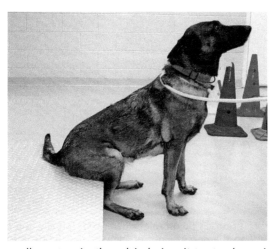

Fig. 8. Sitting on a small step to raise the pelvis during sit-to-stand exercises. (*From* Millis DL, Drum M, Levine D. Therapeutic exercises: joint motion, strengthening, endurance, and speed exercises. In: Millis DL, Levine D, Taylor RA, editors. Canine rehabilitation and physical therapy. St Louis (MO): Saunders; 2014. p. 518; with permission.)

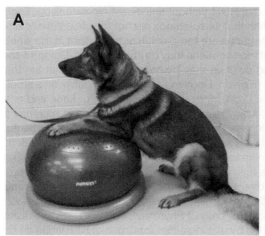
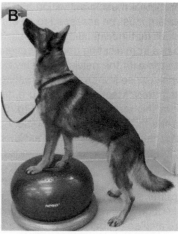

Fig. 9. (A) Advanced sit-to-stand exercise using a FitPAWS® Donut and Donut Holder (product permission from Ball Dynamics International, Longmont, CO). (B) This can dramatically increase the difficulty of sit-to-stand exercises and should only be initiated once simple and moderate difficulty sit-to-stands are accomplished with ease.

to crouch to a greater degree as strength and ability allow. Repetitions of 10 to 20 are a general starting point. As the exercise progresses, patients can perform alternating under-over movements with the limbo pole.

Circling, Figure-of-Eight Walking, Vertical Weave Poles

Circling aids in lateral flexion of the spine, strengthening of adductor and abductor muscles, balance, and proprioception. Figure-of-eight walking is a progression of

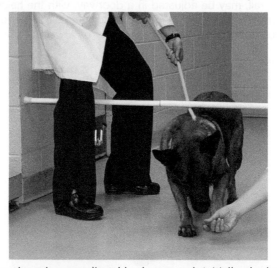

Fig. 10. Limbo exercise using an adjustable shower rod. Initially, the height of the pole should be just lower than the dog's height at the withers. The height should be reduced over time, and the pole heights should be recorded in the patient's chart. (*From* Millis DL, Drum M, Levine D. Therapeutic exercises: joint motion, strengthening, endurance, and speed exercises. In: Millis DL, Levine D, Taylor RA, editors. Canine rehabilitation and physical therapy. St Louis (MO): Saunders; 2014. p. 514; with permission.)

circling. It adds additional challenges by changing directions repeatedly and helps to prepare the patient for irregular turning as the patient returns to more normal function. Weaving between vertical poles also helps to promote side bending of the dog's trunk and also challenges proprioceptive functioning and strengthening of limb abductor and adductor muscles, with more sudden changes in direction.

Exercise design

The size of the circles for circling should be large to begin with, and as limb use and proprioception improve, the size of the circles may become smaller. The same principles apply for figure-of-eight walking and weave pole widths. Weave pole widths may be at or slightly larger than the patient's body length initially, but this width can be consistently shortened with each session as tolerated. Circle and figure-of-eight diameter is widely variable depending on patient size, but is approximately five times the body length.

The handler must lead the patient so that the head, neck, and body actually flex as the poles or circles are negotiated. Additional obstacles or differing surfaces can be added for challenges, and may be combined with daily walks using natural obstacles for weave markers.

Alternatively, an advanced version is to have the patient weave between the handler's legs, usually following a treat or toy (such as a Frisbee). The handler can then walk forward and backward while the patient continues to weave through the handler's legs. The patient should be released from exercise restrictions before performing this advanced exercise.

Aquatic Exercises

The most commonly used aquatic exercises are swimming and UWTM walking. Aquatic exercises have specific properties that make them beneficial in a larger number of situations, such as buoyancy, hydrostatic pressure, resistance (viscosity), and surface tension, which result in improved strength, cardiorespiratory and muscular endurance, ROM, and overall well-being.

Research into canine aquatic therapy has demonstrated that specific changes in joint kinematics and weight bearing occur with swimming and UWTM. Weight bearing can be reduced to 38% of body weight in the rear limbs with the water at the height of the greater trochanter.[9] Regarding kinematics, swimming causes greater overall ROM of the stifle but less stifle extension compared with land treadmill walking. In normal dogs, swimming increases pelvic limb overall ROM and individual joint flexion compared with walking, but less extension of all joints compared with walking. The same was true except hip ROM was not affected in postoperative cruciate ligament repair dogs compared with walking. Unfortunately, no data exist for forelimb movement in dogs while swimming. Based on observations, similar increases in flexion and overall ROM would be expected. However, because most dogs use their forelimbs primarily to generate forward movement while swimming, there may be an increased work load on the shoulder, elbow, and carpus. Therefore, specific conditions may benefit from swimming over UWTM treadmill, and vice versa.

UWTM kinematics are of importance when designing exercise programs. In contrast to swimming, joint extension was no different when the water level was at or below the level of the stifle. However, when the water was filled to the greater trochanter, there was less extension of the pelvic limb joints during the propulsion phase of the gait cycle. This is important, because this may make walking in the UWTM more comfortable for dogs with severe hip and stifle osteoarthritis where full extension is often painful. Joint flexion during UWTM walking is greatest when the water level is at or slightly above the target joint. This is of particular importance because each condition may benefit or be negatively impacted, depending on the condition. For example, after elbow arthroscopy for removal of a fragmented medial coronoid process, maintaining normal elbow flexion is a primary goal, and thus the UWTM water level is ideally set at or just above the elbow. In contrast, patients with biceps tendinitis or medial shoulder instability may be worsened if the water level is set at or slightly above the shoulder, because increased flexion could excessively stress injured tissues. In these shoulder cases, the water level should be significantly higher (2 cm or greater) than the point of the shoulder and the speed of the treadmill belt should be very slow when initiating UWTM exercise.

Exercise design

Initial training is similar to land treadmill training, but is often easier because the patient is contained and cannot jump off the treadmill. Even dogs with a history of near drowning incidents or who are fearful of water can be trained to the UWTM. This is likely because the water fills slowly, is most often warm (29–32°C/85–90°F), and the patient's joints are always in a weight-bearing position. For fearful dogs, it is useful to increase confidence by walking into the UWTM chamber without closing the door initially. Many newer units even have double doors, so the patient can walk through the treadmill. Ramps to enter and exit the chamber are also strongly recommended, because even a small step up into the treadmill can prove difficult for many patients. Alternatively, some UWTM units may be recessed in relation to floor level so that they are flush with the floor. It is also of note that many patients jump up in an attempt to escape (because they cannot simply jump off as with land treadmills), and it is important to prevent this behavior because many UWTM patients are restricted from jumping postoperatively. Another evasive behavior is learning to stand with one or multiple feet on the nonmoving edges of the UWTM. Some units come with floating bumpers or removable sloped inserts to prevent standing on the nonmoving sides (**Fig. 11**). Another useful method to prevent cheating is to use foam pool noodles as bumpers. These are advantageous because they can be used not only to prevent standing on the sides, but also standing on the front. Another option is a bar or rope across the top of the UWTM to hook a harness onto, to prevent charging the front or drifting to the rear. Most dogs learn to walk effortlessly on the belt area without bumpers after just a few sessions.

Determining the speed of the UWTM depends on the goals of the UWTM. For example, a slower speed is better for encouraging weight bearing and hip extension

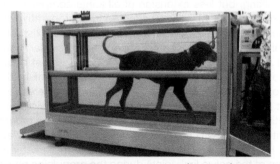

Fig. 11. Plastic bumpers in an UWTM to prevent standing on the nonmoving sides of the UWTM. (*From* Levine D, Millis DL, Flocker J, et al. Aquatic therapy. In: Millis DL, Levine D, Taylor RA, editors. Canine rehabilitation and physical therapy. St Louis (MO): Saunders; 2014. p. 532; with permission.)

in femoral head and neck excision cases, whereas a faster speed is better for muscular and cardiovascular challenge in conditioning obese or athletic dogs. However, the ideal speed may not be the same for every dog within the same condition. The speed should be adjusted such that affected limb use is maximized, but lameness does not increase. Therefore, it is paramount that the patient's gait be monitored at all times and adjustments to the UWTM parameters be made dynamically. Common speeds used for initial UWTM are between 0.3 and 0.5 m/s (0.7 and 1.1 mph) for medium to large dogs. Dachshunds most often need to begin between 0.18 and 0.25 m/s (0.4 and 0.6 mph), given their chondrodystrophic stature. Other small and toy breeds often walk comfortably between 0.2 and 0.3 m/s (0.5 and 0.7 mph). The speed for the first UWTM session is often much slower than the subsequent sessions because there is always some trepidation during the first session. There is no perfect duration of time for every patient, but the authors frequently use intervals for the first several sessions, particularly in deconditioned patients. For example, a standard cruciate repair would begin with the water level at the level of the flank, a speed of 0.36 and 0.45 m/s (0.8–1.0 mph) and duration of 2 minutes, repeated three times with 2-minute rest intervals. However, the time is determined by the success of the training period. A dog that requires many short durations of training would not complete a full interval course. Some dogs only complete the initial UWTM acclimation training during the first UWTM session. Once an ideal speed has been determined, increases to the duration of UWTM walking are made every one or two sessions, with a goal of 20 to 30 minutes of continuous walking in most cases. Speed changes are made as needed depending on the condition. For example, a cruciate repair case may be held at the same speed for the first 3 weeks of therapy until limb use and strength is consistent without any exercise-induced lameness. Then, the patient may have the UWTM speed increased every session and further advanced to interval speeds over a 15- to 20-minute-long session, in addition to other therapeutic exercises within the outpatient session.

Additional aids, such as inflatable water wings, resistance bands, life vests, water weights, boots, or resistance jets, can be used for perturbation or increased challenge in aquatic therapy (**Fig. 12**). They are most successful with UWTM exercise. Swimming provides an increased challenge to the cardiorespiratory system; many weak or debilitated patients require assistance during swimming. During an assisted swim, the therapist can also provide additional perturbation by rolling the patient to stimulate a righting reflex, and create resistance to or assist with limb movements. Most pools have stair steps for entry and exit and these can be used not only as a rest station,

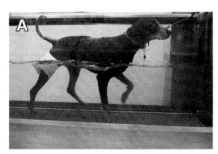 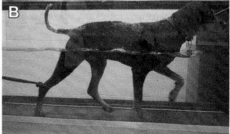

Fig. 12. Use of a water wing (*A*) and resistance band (*B*) to increase ROM and resistance during UWTM exercise. (*From* Millis DL, Drum M, Levine D. Therapeutic exercises: joint motion, strengthening, endurance, and speed exercises. In: Millis DL, Levine D, Taylor RA, editors. Canine rehabilitation and physical therapy. St Louis (MO): Saunders; 2014. p. 522; with permission.)

but for the therapist to perform passive ROM or weight-shifting exercises during an assisted swim to be more efficient with the aquatic session. Even dogs that readily swim in lakes, ponds, or other bodies of water can be trained to an individual pool where they can swim in a constrained space and under controlled conditions, compared with lakes and ponds. Additionally, many dogs are unfamiliar with using stairs to enter and exit a pool, so training should initially be focused on reducing stress on entry, learning to remain in the pool, and exiting on command. Patients should wear a personal flotation device (life vest) when being introduced to swimming not only as a safety measure, but also to provide a handle to guide the patient during swim training. A life vest with a broad abdominal support is preferred to provide maximal comfort (**Fig. 13**). If after two or three training sessions the patient is still stressed, swimming may not be a good choice of exercise for that particular patient. Similarly, if the patient does not use the affected limb in the desired manner, another exercise should be substituted. However, a patient with multiple problems, such as an obese Labrador Retriever recovering from tibial plateau leveling osteotomy surgery, benefits from swimming for the aerobic activity despite potential poor limb use, compared with UWTM or land-based exercises.

Leg Weights and Resistance Bands

The therapist can increase resistance to a particular limb or muscle group using a leg weight or elastic resistance band (**Fig. 14**). Many leg weights designed for people do not fit properly. Human leg weights are often far too heavy, too large, and difficult to maintain in the desired position. Placement of the weight on the limb should also be considered. The stress on the limb is less when the weight is placed closer to the affected limb segment. A general rule of thumb is to use a weight that ranges between 1% and 3% of body weight, depending on limb strength and the stage of recovery. Leg weights are most effective in strengthening flexor muscles, which can be difficult to target with most active exercises. Additionally, the flexor muscles eventually fatigue and the limb is gradually lowered to the ground. This may be beneficial in difficult non–weight-bearing cases, such as some femoral head and neck excisions.

Elastic resistance bands are also frequently used for limb muscle strengthening. Bands come in various degrees of resistance. There are many ways to use an elastic

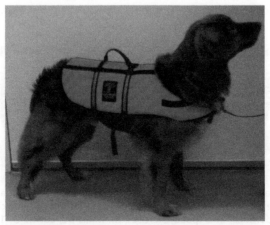

Fig. 13. Canine lifejacket. Note the broad abdominal band supporting the thorax and abdomen. This design is preferred over simple nylon straps.

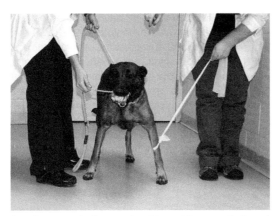

Fig. 14. Resistance band use to challenge shoulder adductors during therapeutic exercise. (*From* Millis DL, Drum M, Levine D. Therapeutic exercises: joint motion, strengthening, endurance, and speed exercises. In: Millis DL, Levine D, Taylor RA, editors. Canine rehabilitation and physical therapy. St Louis (MO): Saunders; 2014. p. 521; with permission.)

band to increase the contraction strength of a specific muscle group. A common method is to secure the band to the involved extremity as the handler provides resistance on the opposite end. For example, while walking on a ground treadmill, lateral tension is applied to the band, so that the adductor muscles must contract to a greater degree. Another method is to use a harness to attach the bands while performing specific exercises, such as side stepping. Resistance bands may also be used in aquatic exercises, and in these situations, the band should be stretched out and dried flat after the exercise to avoid sticking together and degrading. When introducing resistance to an exercise, begin with 50% of the duration and repetitions with resistance. Thus, if performing 20 repetitions of side stepping, add resistance to 10 out of 20 repetitions or limit to 10 repetitions all with resistance. When performing in combination, initially focus on walking slowly with resistance and rapidly without. Progress to increasing the speed of the activity as the patient improves.

Controlled Ball Playing

Ball playing is a fun and effective form of therapeutic exercise that dogs and their owners enjoy. It also has the potential to cause damage to surgical repairs. Controlled activity is the key. The degree of activity depends on the surgical procedure performed, the condition of the tissues, and the stage of tissue healing. In the early postoperative period, ball playing should be indoors in a small room or on a relatively short leash to avoid explosive activity. As the patient progresses, the dog graduates to ball playing in an enclosed area, such as a run. As the animal nears full return to function, off-leash activity may be performed in a large fenced field free of irregular surfaces. The main benefits of ball playing are to increase power, speed, and muscle strength. In most conditions, jumping should be avoided to reduce the risk of injury. It is important to start by rolling the ball or throwing such that the ball is not bouncing high in the air, which encourages jumping.

SUMMARY

Therapeutic exercises to increase active ROM, strength, endurance, speed, and proprioception are the cornerstone of any rehabilitation program. Combining therapeutic exercise with manual techniques and other modalities is the best approach to achieve maximal function. The rehabilitation team, including the owner or handler, is only limited by their resourcefulness and imagination. Therapeutic exercise programs should be tailored to the specific activities the patient is expected to perform, but the patient may need to begin with low-level activities before progressing to higher-level activities. Variety is essential to prevent the owner and patient from becoming bored and allowing appropriate progression of load and tissues. Exercise programs should be designed so that all involved tissues are challenged for strengthening, but not so rapidly as to result in complications and tissue damage. Finally, therapeutic exercise should be fun and interesting for the therapist, the owner, and most importantly the patient.

REFERENCES

1. Augustsson J, Esko A, Thomeé R, et al. Weight training of the thigh muscles using closed vs. open kinetic chain exercises: a comparison of performance enhancement. J Orthop Sports Phys Ther 1998;27:3–8.
2. McArdle WD, Katch FI, Katch VL. Muscular strength: training muscles to become stronger. In: Exercise physiology: nutrition, energy, and human performance, 22, 7th edition. Philadelphia: Lippincott Williams & Wilkins; 2010. p. 490–528.
3. Thorn JM, Templeton JJ, Van Winkle KM, et al. Conditioning shelter dogs to sit. J Appl Anim Welf Sci 2006;9:25–39.
4. Holler PJ, Brazda V, Dal-Bianco B. Kinematic motion analysis of the joints of the forelimbs and hind limbs of dogs during walking exercise regimens. Am J Vet Res 2010;71:734–40.
5. Millis DL, Levine D. Canine rehabilitation and physical therapy. Philadelphia: Saunders; 2014.
6. Carr J, Millis DL, Weng HY. Exercises in canine physical rehabilitation: range of motion of the forelimb during stair and ramp ascent. J Small Anim Pract 2013; 54:409–13.
7. Durant AM, Millis DL, Headrick FJ. Kinematics of stair ascent in healthy dogs. Vet Comp Orthop Traumatol 2011;24:99–105.
8. Feeney LC, Lin CF, Marcellin-Little DJ, et al. Validation of two-dimensional kinematic analysis of walk and sit-to-stand motions in dogs. Am J Vet Res 2007;68: 277–82.
9. Levine D, Marcellin-Little DJ, Millis DL, et al. Effects of partial immersion on vertical ground reaction forces and weight distribution in dogs. Am J Vet Res 2010;71:1413–6.

Rehabilitation and Physical Therapy for Selected Orthopedic Conditions in Veterinary Patients

Andrea L. Henderson, DVM, CCRP[a], Christian Latimer, DVM[b],
Darryl L. Millis, MS, DVM, DACVS, CCRP, DACVSMR[b],*

KEYWORDS

- Tendon • Ligament • Shoulder • Muscle • Orthopedic conditions

KEY POINTS

- A specific diagnosis is needed to perform optimal rehabilitation of orthopedic problems.
- A comprehensive rehabilitation plan is particularly important for orthopedic patients when surgical repairs are mechanically weak, for examples when repairing fractures in skeletally immature patients or when repairing tendons or ligaments.
- Joint immobilization is used to protect weak surgical repairs. The duration of immobilization should be minimized, particularly in situations with potential loss of joint motion.
- Evidence-based information regarding specific modalities and techniques for rehabilitation of injured dogs and cats is limited. The choice of modalities and techniques must be based on common sense and clinical experience.

Rehabilitation and physical therapy for patients with orthopedic conditions are common. Although rehabilitation of several conditions has been described in detail, rehabilitation of less common conditions may be challenging. This article provides information regarding some of these conditions, including articular and periarticular fractures, shoulder conditions, muscle conditions, tendon and ligament injuries, and osteoarthritis (OA).

REHABILITATION OF ARTICULAR AND PERIARTICULAR FRACTURES

Articular and periarticular fractures occur relatively commonly in veterinary patients, and these fractures carry specific risks because of loss of joint or physeal integrity.

[a] Joint Base San Antonio, Lackland, San Antonio, Texas 78236, USA; [b] Department of Small Animal Clinical Sciences, College of Veterinary Medicine, University of Tennessee, 2407 River Drive, Knoxville, TN 37996, USA
* Corresponding author.
E-mail address: dmillis@utk.edu

Vet Clin Small Anim 45 (2015) 91–121
http://dx.doi.org/10.1016/j.cvsm.2014.09.006
0195-5616/15/$ – see front matter © 2015 Elsevier Inc. All rights reserved.

Possible sequelae to fractures causing disruption of the articular surface or damage to the growth plate include abnormal bone growth, development of OA, and performance and mobility deficits. Early goals of rehabilitation for articular and periarticular fractures include maintaining or improving joint and segment range of motion (ROM), providing pain relief, minimizing periarticular fibrosis, and giving sufficient time for bone healing by allowing progressive loading that will prevent implant failure and will augment, rather than disrupt, bone healing. After sufficient healing has occurred to support partial physiologic loads, the rehabilitation program should include exercises to promote muscle and bone strengthening, continued improvement of ROM, and gradual return to activities of sport/daily living.[1]

Articular Fractures

Rigid fixation and anatomic reduction of articular fractures are critical operative goals to optimize joint function and reduce or prevent osteoarthritic progression. However, surgical repair cannot completely address musculoskeletal tissues surrounding the fracture that are critical for physiologic movement and ROM. Periarticular musculoskeletal tissues are damaged by the original injury, and surgical repair induces additional damage to these periarticular tissues because extensive debridement and soft tissue disruption may be necessary to achieve the desired articular cartilage alignment and fragment reduction to maximize long-term joint health.[2] Recent advances in surgery have led to increased emphasis on minimally invasive techniques to reduce soft tissue manipulation, incorporating the assistance of arthroscopy or fluoroscopy to ensure adequate fragment reduction and articular alignment.[3,4] The rehabilitation plan must take the biomechanics of the repair method into consideration to prevent excessive loading and disruption of fragments, joints, or implants, while minimizing loss of associated musculoskeletal soft tissue integrity and function.

Physeal Fractures

Growth plates in skeletally immature patients have the highest risk of disruption with excessive stress or trauma. The hypertrophic zone of chondrocytes is particularly susceptible to damage in response to compressive or shearing forces.[3] Disruption of cellular maturation, through either direct or indirect trauma, can lead to decreased limb length and/or angular limb deformities as the patient continues to grow.[5] Physeal fractures are typically described using the Salter-Harris classification system, numbered according to increasing severity.

Salter-Harris type I: The fracture involves only the physis.

Salter-Harris type II: The fracture involves the physis and the metaphysis.

Salter-Harris type III: The fracture involves the physis and the epiphysis, with disruption of the articular surface.

Salter-Harris type IV: The fracture involves the physis and extends into both the metaphysis and the epiphysis.

Salter-Harris type V: This category describes a compressive force causing a fracture and collapse of part or all of the physis, causing premature closure and a potential for abnormal growth and/or angular limb deformities.

Physeal fractures in young animals generally do not involve multiple articular fragments as often occurs in mature patients with articular fractures. However, they present their own unique challenges for postoperative rehabilitation because of the rapid and exuberant healing response, and the potential for premature closure of the physis, especially with crushing trauma to the physis. Initial repair and correction of angular limb deformities after premature closure of a physis must be timed accordingly for a patient population that heals rapidly and demonstrates continual long bone growth.

Soft bone in young patients must be handled carefully during and after surgery, and implants are often located in areas with small fragments and are therefore intrinsically weaker. Young patients additionally tend to have an increased activity level and lower tolerance for rehabilitation techniques, such as passive ROM (PROM) and stretching, that may cause mild discomfort in the early postoperative period.[2] For these reasons, some surgeons have immobilized limbs in extension during the early postoperative period to reduce load-bearing and risk of implant failure. However, loss of ROM accompanied by soft tissue fibrosis and/or contracture is a severe complication associated with immobilization, along with atrophy and cartilage degeneration.[1] Therefore, alternative techniques should be considered to reduce weight-bearing that preserves ROM.

Common articular and physeal fractures in veterinary patients include Salter-Harris type II fractures of the distal femur, Salter-Harris type I femoral capital physeal fractures, and Salter-Harris type IV fractures of the lateral aspect of the humeral condyle.

Distal Femoral Fractures

Distal fractures represent 20% to 25% of femoral fractures in veterinary patients.[6] These injuries occur most often in puppies between 4 and 11 months of age and are most commonly Salter-Harris type II fractures.[2,3,6] Only a small percentage (17%) involves the articular surface of the stifle[6] and these most often involve both femoral condyles.[7] Surgical repair within 48 hours of injury facilitates anatomic reduction and may improve the postoperative prognosis. In addition, early postoperative rehabilitation is a critical factor in managing these fractures to prevent contracture of the quadriceps muscle. Quadriceps contracture, also known as "quadriceps tie-down," is a potentially devastating postoperative complication of distal femoral physeal fracture repair. Damage to the quadriceps muscle leads to fibrosis and scar tissue formation with subsequent adhesion to the distal femur, preventing normal function of the quadriceps muscle and stifle extension. Historically, some surgeons have elected to limit load-bearing during the early postoperative period by splinting the limb in extension.[8] Immobilization in extension for as little as 5 to 7 days after surgery is sufficient to allow quadriceps contracture to begin.[1] Quadriceps contracture can also occur without immobilization, as a complication of limb disuse.[8] In addition to contracture of the muscle, muscle atrophy, loss of bone mass, and articular and periarticular fibrosis can occur as sequelae of immobilization. Tissue damage may reach sufficient severity to result in genu recurvatum, ankylosis of the stifle joint, and a nonfunctional limb.[1,9] Therefore, to prevent complications of splinting or bandaging the limb with the stifle in extension, the authors prefer to place a 90-90 flexion sling on the limb immediately after surgery to maintain the quadriceps muscle and cranial joint capsule in a stretched position for at least overnight following surgery (**Fig. 1**). Most patients will be treated with postoperative analgesics and sedation and will have swelling and discomfort following surgery. Most puppies will be uncomfortable immediately after surgery and unwilling to use the limb, so this is a good time to provide passive prolonged stretching of the tissues until pain and swelling are under control.

The initial physical rehabilitation program for distal femoral fracture repairs should include cryotherapy followed by gentle massage to reduce swelling. Cryotherapy and initial massage may begin while the patient is recovering from anesthesia. Before complete recovery from anesthesia, the 90-90 flexion sling is applied. Cryotherapy may be applied 4 to 6 times daily for 20 minutes per session, depending on the degree of swelling and edema. After 72 hours, cryotherapy can be exchanged for heat therapy if clinical evidence of inflammation is adequately reduced. Passive ROM of all joints of the affected limb, and stifle flexion stretches with 15- to 30-second holds, should be

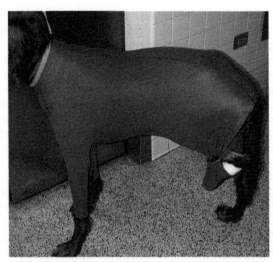

Fig. 1. A body sock used as a 90-90 flexion sling to maintain the stifle in a flexed position following surgery for a distal femoral fracture.

performed 3 to 6 times daily. In addition, gentle weight-shifting exercises and sling-assisted walking to encourage limb use are appropriate in the early postoperative period. The 90-90 stifle flexion sling may be applied for the first 2 to 3 days after surgery if the dog is weight-bearing on the limb or to limit uncontrolled weight-bearing.[1] However, the device should be removable to allow for several therapeutic sessions daily. Within 10 to 14 days after surgery, the active program can progress to gentle tug-of-war and leaning exercises, low Cavaletti rails to encourage stifle flexion, more challenging weight-shifting on unstable surfaces, and underwater treadmill therapy after the incision has sealed. Swimming is an effective exercise after fracture healing has progressed sufficiently (2–3 weeks) to allow low-load ROM in patients that use their pelvic limbs in the water. However, caution must be exercised to limit vigorous movements against the resistance of the water until radiographic bone union has occurred. In general, these fractures heal very quickly, usually within 3 to 4 weeks. If at any time limb use suddenly deteriorates, radiographs should be made to be certain that there are no signs of infection and fixation failure has not occurred. The authors like to maintain the patient in the hospital for rehabilitation until ROM is relatively pain-free and moderate weight-bearing occurs on the limb. Most patients are discharged within 1 to 4 days after surgery. Patients are followed very closely in the first 2 weeks to be certain that quadriceps contracture is not occurring. Treatment of early quadriceps contracture is relatively successful, but after the contracture has mature fibrous tissue, it is a much more difficult problem to manage and the prognosis is more guarded, often requiring surgery and intensive in-house physical rehabilitation for several weeks.

If quadriceps contracture occurs, treatment may be attempted with surgical debridement and breakdown of the scar tissue adhesions, followed by an intense physical rehabilitation program to maintain restored ROM and prevent reoccurrence of the adhesions. Adhesions of the quadriceps muscle to the femur are surgically released. Release of certain aspects of the joint capsule and other tissues may also be necessary. A 90-90 flexion sling is applied for several days after surgery, with removal of the device 4 to 6 times daily for rehabilitation. Normal ROM and limb use were achieved with quadriceps adhesion release, temporary placement of a static stifle flexion apparatus, and intense physical therapy in a 4-month-old golden retriever puppy suffering from quadriceps contracture after failed repair of a comminuted femoral diaphyseal fracture.[8] Prevention of quadriceps contracture carries a much better prognosis than treatment after it has already occurred. All patients with distal femoral fracture repairs should be repaired as soon as possible after injury if the patient is stable, and surgery should be performed with minimally invasive techniques to reduce the amount of periosteal reaction, scar tissue formation, and adhesion. In addition, patients should receive a physical rehabilitation program that focuses initially on alleviation of pain, early controlled limb use, and preservation of ROM with a focus on stifle flexion and hip extension.

Proximal Femoral Fractures

Proximal femoral fractures typically occur at the femoral capital physis in young animals and at the femoral neck in mature animals. The flattened surfaces of the proximal femoral physis render it prone to shear forces; therefore, most fractures are of the Salter-Harris type I category.[5] Fractures involving the articular surface of the hip are rare, given the relatively protected position of the head of the femur within the acetabulum and the biomechanics of weight-bearing. Capital physeal fractures are especially concerning in puppies less than 5 months of age with large growth potential. The aftermath of these fractures can include premature closure of the physis, a shortened femoral neck, and decreased femoral head size despite anatomic reduction with internal fixation, leading to hip incongruity and degenerative joint disease beginning in early adulthood.

Surgical repair of capital physeal fractures commonly includes a combination of screws placed in lag fashion and/or divergent Kirschner wires. Postoperative muscle contracture is not typically a concern in this area as it is with distal femoral fractures, given the small epiphyseal segment involved. However, some surgeons may elect to immobilize cases for 1 to 2 weeks postoperatively with an Ehmer sling; therefore, ROM preservation remains a concern. Removal of the sling should take place as early as possible for rehabilitation sessions, including cryotherapy and PROM. Active ROM can also be achieved with early weight-bearing exercises, such as balance and weight-shifting, slow leash-walking including declines, and low Cavaletti rails. Later exercises when more physiologic loads are acceptable include underwater treadmill walking, swimming, incline walking, slow stair climbing, and backwards walking. Beginning at 4 to 5 weeks after a stable repair, the program can include activities at higher speeds, walking through sand or snow, and dancing to encourage hind limb propulsion and hamstring and gluteal muscle activity. Postoperative radiographs should be obtained to evaluate healing and hip congruity at 4 weeks before accelerating the program.

Postoperative complications include infection, avascular necrosis due to disruption of blood supply to the femoral head, loss of anatomic reduction, and implant penetration into the joint.[1,5,6] The therapist should monitor for crepitus, increased pain, or loss of ROM. In cases in which early surgical repair, adequate reduction, or prevention of hip incongruity cannot be achieved, femoral head and neck excision or total hip replacement may provide long-term relief of pain. Prognosis for femoral capital physeal fracture fixation is improved with early repair (48–72 hours after injury), increased patient age, and decreased soft tissue damage.[5]

Humeral Condylar Fractures

Fractures of the lateral aspect of the humeral condyle are by far the most common fractures of the elbow in dogs and are typically of the Salter-Harris type IV category in skeletally immature dogs. However, distal humeral fractures in adult dogs as a result of repetitive concussive forces along with incomplete intracondylar ossification are recognized in a growing number of breeds. Among the most common breeds represented are cocker spaniels and English Springer spaniels, but a predisposition has also been observed in Labrador retrievers and Rottweilers.[10,11] Although the lateral aspect of the condyle is most commonly affected, bicondylar or "Y" fractures are also relatively common, with fractures involving only the medial aspect of the condyle along with the physis less commonly. One study[12] found a case distribution of 56%, 33%, and 11% for the 3 affected regions, respectively. These proportions may be explained by the fact that most of the biomechanical forces are transmitted from the radius to the capitulum on the lateral aspect of the humeral condyle during weight-bearing. In addition, the lateral portion is thinner and weaker than its medial counterpart which makes it more susceptible to bending in forces in response to weight-bearing.[13]

Surgical repair of humeral condylar fractures includes placement of a transcondylar screw in lag fashion to provide compression across the condyle, along with an antirotational pin across the affected metaphyseal fractured segment or segments. In large breeds or working dogs, plating the epicondylar surface may be most appropriate to counteract expected forces. Complication rates for lateral condylar fractures have been reported to be 15% to 35%.[12,13] Considerably higher postoperative complication rates (46%–64%) are reported for bicondylar fractures.[14–16] However, better outcomes and lower complication rates have been seen when medial and lateral exposures were made rather than the more common historical practice of performing an olecranon osteotomy to allow access from a single approach.[17] Outcomes can be very satisfactory after surgical repair of humeral condylar fractures with appropriate stabilization and postoperative management. A retrospective evaluation found that 44% of 16 farm working dogs returned to excellent function and 50% returned to their duties with some limitations, although one-third of the operated dogs had postoperative complications requiring a second surgery.[13] However, long-term risk of degenerative joint disease is high; one study[18] found that OA developed in all of 15 dogs with humeral condylar fractures with median follow-up time of 43 months after surgery. Functional and clinical outcome appear not to be associated with the accuracy of articular fracture reduction.[17,18] However, a recent retrospective study found that complication rate increased with screw placement angled dorsoventrally as it traversed through the condyle where the ideal position (zero degrees) was considered parallel with a line passing through the lateral and medial humeral epicondyles.[12] Appropriate physical rehabilitation with control of weight-bearing forces and ROM contribute substantially to the prognosis for recovery of function.

In the early postoperative inflammatory period, physical rehabilitation should consist of cryotherapy, pain relief, massage, PROM, and gentle weight-shifting exercises with assistance. If sufficient concern about the stability of the repair warrants prevention of weight-bearing for several weeks, use of a carpal flexion bandage is recommended over a sling, when possible, to preserve elbow ROM. In addition, carpal and digital extension exercises should be performed routinely at bandage changes. ROM exercises should be performed for 3 to 4 weeks after surgery, despite early clinical improvement, allowing periarticular fibrous tissues to mature.[1] Passive ROM exercises should be performed by a professional for the first 2 to 3 weeks after injury, because a fine balance point exists between adequate end ranges and excessive force.[1] The therapist is urged to exercise extreme caution in the early rehabilitation of very young dogs with Salter-Harris fractures of the humeral condyle. The bones are extremely soft, and it is common for the implants to loosen and back out, resulting in loss of reduction and joint apposition if rehabilitation is too vigorous. In general, PROM, weight shifting, and limited controlled leash walking may be used 2 to 4 times daily, with crate rest in-between. Puppies often want to jump and play, and this should be avoided. If healing is progressing as expected, active ROM exercises such as light paw-shaking, easy tug-of-war, and rolling slowly forward and backward with the antebrachii resting on a therapy roll may begin 3 weeks after surgery (**Fig. 2**). After 3 to 4 weeks, gentle underwater treadmill walking, swimming, Cavaletti rails, and inclines can be used. If progressing well and there is radiographic evidence of adequate healing, patients can then participate in exercises with resistance weights on the distal limb and more rigorous stair and obstacle navigation activities.

Additional Articular and Periarticular Fractures

The most common articular and periarticular fractures of veterinary patients have been discussed above. However, additional uncommon fractures involving the joints or physes include avulsion of the supraglenoid tubercle, carpal and tarsal fractures, quadriceps (patella) or tibial tuberosity avulsion fractures, and fractures of the proximal humeral, tibial, radial, or ulnar physes.

Supraglenoid tubercle avulsion fractures may occasionally occur in immature animals. The supraglenoid tubercle is typically displaced distally, due to the force generated by concentric contraction of the biceps brachii muscle.[3] Larger fragments may be repaired, but fragment removal and effective biceps release are alternative options. In the case of fragment repair of other articular fractures involving the glenoid cavity, non-weight-bearing slings are often used to immobilize the limb postoperatively due to large weight-bearing forces on relatively small fragments of the shoulder joint.[1] Ideally, a commercial sling is used that can be removed for physical rehabilitation, including massage, PROM, and cryotherapy or heat therapy as indicated. Exercises that promote strengthening of the biceps brachii and/or brachialis can be initiated after sufficient fracture healing has occurred to allow weight-bearing forces. Examples of such exercises include paw-shaking with the gradual addition of resistance weights, wheelbarrowing forward and backward, swimming, and pushups on a therapy roll.

Carpal and tarsal fractures have historically been most common in racing greyhounds possibly contributed by asymmetric bone remodeling based on the stresses incurred during repetitive counterclockwise sprinting. The most common carpal bones to fracture in these sporting dogs are the radial and accessory carpal bones.

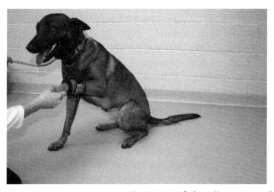

Fig. 2. Shake paws exercise to encourage active ROM of the elbow joint following repair of a fracture of the lateral portion of the humeral condyle.

Most non-sporting-dog carpal and tarsal fractures occur in association with trauma such as motor vehicle accidents, with forces sufficient to cause extensive tissue damage. Fractures may be repaired with screws or pins if the piece is large enough. Small fragments may simply be removed. Often, carpal or tarsal arthrodesis is used as a salvage procedure in cases of extensive fracture. Physical rehabilitation techniques for carpal and tarsal fracture repairs are similar to those in use with other articular fractures, including early analgesia, ROM, and partial weight-bearing, with progressive increase of load during active exercises. External coaptation is necessary for 6 to 8 weeks following a carpal or tarsal arthrodesis to allow early bone formation; the therapist should focus on ROM of the nonfused joints during bandage changes. Following removal of external coaptation, progressive weight-bearing, gait-retraining, and exercises that promote muscle hypertrophy and active ROM can begin.[1]

Physical rehabilitation of articular and periarticular fractures in veterinary patients requires a thorough understanding of their unique surgical challenges and potential postoperative complications. Rigid fixation, anatomic reduction, and minimal soft tissue disruption are well-understood as important operative principles in the management of these types of fractures. In addition, the physical rehabilitation program is a key contributor to a good outcome for articular and periarticular fractures by providing early ROM, soft tissue mobilization, atrophy reduction, and safe, progressive return to function.

PHYSICAL THERAPY AND REHABILITATION FOR SELECTED SHOULDER DISORDERS

Shoulder conditions are increasingly recognized as a source of lameness and dysfunction, especially in sporting and working dogs. The use of MRI, diagnostic ultrasound, and diagnostic arthroscopy has greatly aided the specific diagnosis of shoulder conditions.

Bicipital Tenosynovitis

Conservative management and rehabilitation for bicipital tenosynovitis in dogs involve stabilization and stretching exercises, and restriction from strenuous exercise. Cryotherapy, therapeutic ultrasound, therapeutic laser (light amplification by stimulated emission of radiation),[19] and extracorporeal shock-wave therapy may also be of benefit, although specific clinical studies have not been performed to evaluate dose, frequency, and efficacy of therapeutic modalities. In addition, nonsteroidal anti-inflammatory drugs (NSAIDs) are also administered in early mild bicipital tenosynovitis.[20] Later stages are frequently treated with intra-articular corticosteroids with reasonable success.[21] Injections are made in the shoulder joint because this joint communicates with the biceps tendon sheath. Recently, biological treatments, such as platelet-rich plasma (PRP) and stem cell therapy, have been advocated. Although the efficacy of these treatments is unknown, anecdotal experience suggests that these treatments may be beneficial in some cases. Severe tendon damage or recurrent bouts of tenosynovitis are often surgically managed with either simple biceps tendon release or release and tenodesis to the proximal humerus.

The initial goals of treatment are to reduce inflammation, pain, and swelling, accomplished with rest, cryotherapy, transcutaneous electrical nerve stimulation (TENS), laser and anti-inflammatory medication. Exercise should be restricted to leash walks only with no running, jumping, or playing until lameness resolves. During the reduced activity period, physical modalities may be instituted. After soundness at a walk returns, a slowly progressive rehabilitation and therapeutic exercise program may be instituted.

The correct region of application of any modality is important. Clinicians frequently treat in an incorrect area, usually on the lateral aspect of the greater tubercle. Review of the anatomy of the biceps tendon and muscle is important.[20] The biceps originates from the supraglenoid tubercle and courses through the intertubercular groove of the humerus, which is located medial to the greater tubercle.

A 3.3-MHz pulsed-mode ultrasound over the tendon and musculotendinous junction during the acute inflammatory phase of the condition provides the biologic effects of ultrasound, such as angiogenesis and fibroblast proliferation, without the thermal effects that may increase inflammation. The intensity of the ultrasound may be 1.5 to 2 W/cm^2 because the pulsed-mode ultrasound should not result in significantly elevated tissue temperature. As the acute phase resolves, continuous-mode ultrasound increases collagen extensibility, pain threshold, blood flow, and macrophage and enzyme activity. This deep heating also helps to decrease muscle spasms that may be present. Because ultrasound waves are reflected to areas in close proximity, such as bone, signs of pain due to excessive tissue temperature increase should be monitored as well.

Extracorporeal shock-wave therapy has also been used in bicipital tenosynovitis patients to decrease inflammation of the tendon and promote healing through increased cell metabolism, release of growth factors, and increased fibrosis.[22] In general, 500 pulses are applied to the area at a medium intensity (0.13 J/cm^2), every 2 weeks.

Therapeutic laser may also be beneficial. Doses of 3 to 9 J/cm^2 several times weekly may be applied, especially for acute cases.[19]

As lameness resolves, gentle ROM to the shoulder joint and cautious stretching of the biceps muscle and tendon may be instituted. Initially, stretching should be limited to flexion of the shoulder only. As the condition improves, and tissue tightness is less apparent, gentle extension of the elbow while flexing the shoulder provides additional stretch to the muscle-tendon unit. The stretch should be less vigorous if any pain or discomfort is elicited.

Deep transverse friction massage is a rehabilitation option for bicipital tenosynovitis after resolution of acute inflammation. This technique may result in mild inflammation, so it is important to perform these manipulations during the more chronic periods of inflammation. The presumption behind this method is that mild, acute controlled inflammation will aid in healing, improve collagen extensibility, and prevent adhesions between structures. Deep frictional massage is applied perpendicular to the fibers for 5 minutes daily during the initial treatment. As the condition becomes more chronic, the massage is applied for 20 minutes, 3 times per week. Deep frictional massage can exacerbate the condition, particularly when performed incorrectly.

Therapeutic exercises initially consist of slow leash walks, 3-legged standing for general limb strengthening, and proprioceptive exercises, such as weight-shifting and balance board activities. General strengthening of the tissues may be instituted with shake hands exercise, Cavaletti rail walking, and walking down a gradual slope. As strength improves, and if there is no return of lameness, other activities may be instituted such as walking with a therapy band on a treadmill with the band resisting elbow flexion, wheelbarrowing, wearing a limb weight while walking over Cavaletti rails, underwater treadmill walking progressing to swimming, standing on a therapy roll or ball, and jogging down inclines. Finally, sport-specific activities may be introduced after 8 to 12 weeks, depending on the severity of the initial injury and the response to treatment.

Supraspinatus Muscle Conditions

Common conditions of the supraspinatus muscle and tendon in dogs include trauma and tearing of tendon fibers, calcification of the tendon, and degeneration of the tendon with core lesion formation. Dogs competing in agility and fly ball events may be at increased risk of injury, with repetitive trauma and stress to the shoulder region causing injury with resultant lameness. Physical diagnosis may be confusing, because concurrent injuries, such as biceps tenosynovitis or medial shoulder injury, may also be present. Direct palpation over the insertion of the tendon on the cranial aspect of the greater tubercle usually elicits pain. Also, adduction of the shoulder joint over the edge of a table with the dog in lateral recumbency and maintaining the shoulder at a standing angle may result in pain. MRI and diagnostic ultrasound are often used to evaluate the area for calcific change to the tendon, core lesions in the tendon, or tearing of tendon fibers.

Biologic treatment is the current preferred method for treatment of core lesions. PRP or stem cells are injected directly into the core lesion under ultrasound guidance. Appropriate rest and exercise restriction are instituted for 8 weeks. During this time, leash walks, PROM, and very cautious stretching may be instituted. Therapeutic laser and ultrasound may also be beneficial during the early phases of healing. Repeat sonograms are recommended at 2 to 4 weeks to assess healing. A second injection may be necessary if an adequate healing response is not seen. Rehabilitation is instituted when initial filling of the core lesion becomes evident. As fibrosis progresses and longitudinal remodeling of fibers occur, additional exercises may be added for strengthening and remodeling of the tendon. Therapeutic exercises initially consist of slow leash walks, 3-legged standing for general limb strengthening, and proprioceptive exercises, such as weight-shifting and balance board activities. General strengthening of the tissues may be instituted with Cavaletti rail walking with the distance between the rails gradually increased over time, and walking up a gradual slope. As strength improves, and if there is no return to pain or lameness, other activities may be instituted, such as walking with a therapy band on a treadmill with the band resisting shoulder extension, wheelbarrowing, underwater treadmill walking progressing to swimming, standing on a therapy roll or ball, and jogging up inclines. Finally, sport-specific activities may be introduced after 10 to 12 weeks, depending on the severity of the initial injury and the response to treatment.

Extracorporeal shock-wave treatment and therapeutic ultrasound may be beneficial for dogs with calcification of the tendon. Surgical removal of calcium deposits has also been described, but conservative treatment may give comparable results and calcification may recur following surgery.[23] Introduction of a rehabilitation program similar to that described for core lesion may be instituted immediately after modalities are applied, and the program may be increased in intensity somewhat sooner because tendon calcification generally indicates a more chronic condition.

Rehabilitation for a partially torn supraspinatus tendon depends on the degree of damage and the stage of healing. Extracorporeal shock-wave treatment, therapeutic laser, and therapeutic ultrasound may all be beneficial in helping with tendon healing. Injection of PRP or stem cells in the affected tendon may also aid healing. As lameness and pain on palpation begin to resolve, rehabilitation similar to that described for core lesions may begin at a rate that does not exacerbate pain and lameness. Careful assessment of the patient at frequent intervals, especially after increasing exercise, is important to prevent setbacks and recurrence of injury.

Fibrotic Contracture of the Infraspinatus Muscle

Fibrotic contracture of the infraspinatus muscle is uncommon and most often affects sporting dogs.[24–27] Lameness typically develops acutely after injury to the infraspinatus tendon and muscle. Over the course of days to weeks, the lameness improves, but a circumducted gait may develop as muscle fibers are replaced with fibrous tissue. After contracture occurs, the treatment of choice is tenotomy of the tendon of insertion of the infraspinatus muscle. This surgery also involves a release of capsular adhesions of the tendon.

In early cases of muscle/tendon injury before contracture occurs, stretching, PROM exercises, targeted therapeutic exercises, ultrasound therapy, therapeutic laser, and extracorporeal shock-wave treatment can help to improve length, mobility, and healing of affected tissues. Physical rehabilitation alone is of little benefit in chronic infraspinatus contracture. It is extremely hard to improve the condition without surgery if severe, chronic contracture is present. After surgery, targeted stretching, frictional massage, and therapeutic exercises are instituted to prevent recurrence of fibrosis and for general muscle strengthening. Often, atrophy of the forelimb muscles occurs with contracture that has been present for more than a month. Conditioning exercises for these muscles, such as walking, jogging, swimming, and wheelbarrowing, should be instituted to allow these muscles to gradually regain their normal size and strength.

Medial Shoulder Instability

The normal shoulder abduction angle for dogs is approximately 30°, whereas dogs with medial shoulder instability (MSI) have abduction angles greater than this with

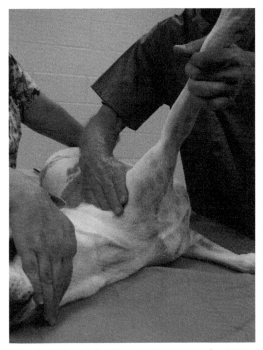

Fig. 3. Evaluation of the shoulder abduction angle to assess for MSI.

pain at the end of abduction (**Fig. 3**).[28] Some dogs with generalized atrophy of the fore-limb muscles may have an increased abduction angle, but there is no pain at the end of abduction. Medial shoulder instability has previously been described as mild, moderate, and severe.[29] Mild and moderate medial glenohumeral instability tends to occur as a result of repetitive physical activity or overuse. Severe instability is less common and usually has a traumatic cause. Instability may be due to stretching or tearing of the medial glenohumeral ligament, subscapularis tendon, joint capsule, or any combination of these.

Patients with mild instability have abduction angles that are 35 to 45° and have mild pathologic changes of the affected shoulder. These dogs generally can be managed conservatively. The authors manage these injuries with extracorporeal shock-wave treatment (750–1000 pulses, 0.14 mJ/cm² initially and then 2 weeks later). After the first treatment, dogs are placed in shoulder hobbles to prevent shoulder abduction for 4 weeks. Rehabilitation should then consist of PROM in a sagittal plane and limited weight-bearing exercises, such as 3-legged standing, balance board exercises, and slow leash walks. Approximately 6 weeks after the start of treatment, other activities can be added, such as light jogging, underwater treadmill walking, and Cavaletti walking. The last phase of therapy is directed at strengthening the muscles, with treadmill walking, while a therapy band is used to put tension on the limb in a lateral direction, causing increased muscle contraction strength of the medial shoulder muscles. Begin with the lightest band and progress every 2 weeks to the next stiffest therapy band.

The range of abduction angles for patients with moderate MSI is 45 to 65°. These dogs have more advanced pathologic abnormalities, such as synovial hyperplasia or hypertrophy, and additional damage to the medial shoulder structures, and will often require biologic therapy and surgical treatment (imbrications, and/or thermal capsulorrhaphy[30]) before physical rehabilitation. The authors have had some success in direct injection of PRP or porcine bladder submucosa in the affected tissues. It may take approximately 3 to 4 months following initial treatment to achieve improved function, and 4 to 6 months for the patient to return to relatively normal function. After

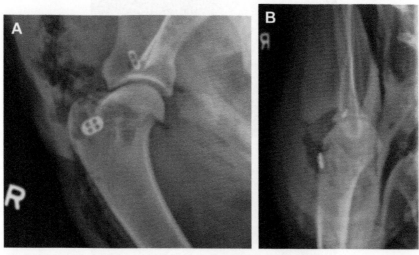

Fig. 4. Postoperative radiographs of a dog after surgical stabilization for MSI. (*A*) Lateral view of shoulder following stabilization. (*B*) Cranial-caudal view of shoulder following stabilization.

surgery, hobbles or a custom shoulder support system should be placed. Cryotherapy and PROM exercises should be instituted for the first 3 weeks. Extracorporeal shock-wave therapy may begin 2 to 4 weeks after surgery. Weight-bearing exercises should be gradually introduced thereafter, similar to that described for mild MSI. If thermal capsulorrhaphy is performed, a non-weight-bearing sling, such as a Velpeau or carpal flexion bandage, is recommended for 4 weeks, followed by hobbles for 2–4 weeks.

Patients are characterized as having severe MSI if their abduction angle is greater than 65°. Complete tears of the medial glenohumeral ligament and pronounced disruption of the subscapularis tendon and joint capsule are often seen during arthroscopic exploration. Severe MSI should be treated with surgical reconstruction, followed by placement of hobbles for 4 weeks (**Fig. 4**). Rehabilitation as described for mild MSI is then initiated, although at a slower rate of progression. Recovery from severe MSI typically takes 5 to 6 months.

Scapular Fractures

Nondisplaced or comminuted fractures of the body of the scapula can often be conservatively managed; however, fractures involving the neck of the scapula or the articular surface of the glenoid typically require open reduction and internal fixation.[29] In either case, the affected shoulder should be held in suspension with a non-weight-bearing sling for 4 to 6 weeks.

Physical rehabilitation is aimed at regaining normal scapular and shoulder motion and includes anti-inflammatory medication, cryotherapy, and PROM exercises targeted at the glenohumeral joint. To limit fibrous tissue formation, cross-fiber frictional massage can be implemented. Scapular glides can be used for increasing ROM. Aquatic therapy and treadmill walking can also be used to attain greater muscle strength. Before exercise, a hot pack can be applied to the affected area to increase extensibility.

Osteochondritis Dissecans of the Humeral Head

Osteochondritis dissecans of the caudal humeral head is the most common developmental shoulder disorder in dogs. The standard treatment is surgical removal of the cartilage flap via arthroscopy or an open arthrotomy, as well as curettage of the bed of the lesion.[29]

For 2 to 4 weeks after surgery, physical rehabilitation includes cryotherapy, PROM exercises, NSAIDS, and short leash walks. More vigorous loading exercises are avoided to allow a period of healing of the lesion with early fibrocartilage formation. Aquatherapy and treadmill walking can be added to the rehabilitation regimen 3 weeks postoperatively. Light jogging can be started at 6 weeks.

REHABILITATION OF MUSCLE CONDITIONS

Muscle conditions are increasingly treated in small animal practice, possibly because of heightened awareness and the increased use of dogs in sporting and working events. Strains of the biceps and supraspinatus muscles may be precursors to more permanent changes to these muscles, described in the section on shoulder conditions. Gracilis, tensor fascia latae, triceps, iliopsoas, gastrocnemius, and biceps muscles are most commonly affected with muscle strains. Muscles that cross 2 joints may be more susceptible to injury because of the greater motion that the muscles must undergo. Strains may occur more commonly in dogs that frequently jump, train in muddy conditions, or pull sleds. Strains are most common in sporting breeds of dogs, and the injury is often not witnessed by the client. Muscle strains may result from forceful contraction of the muscle while the muscle elongates with weight-bearing stress, called eccentric muscle contraction.[31] The patient is presented with a weight-bearing to non-weight-bearing lameness. With mild contusions, there is minimal lameness and the source of pain may be difficult to find. More severe injuries generally have pain and swelling.

Muscle injuries are graded according to severity.[6] Stage 1 injuries indicate mild myositis without disruption of the fascia of myofibrils. Stage 2 injuries are similar to stage 1 but extend to include fascial sheath tears. Stage 3 injury is present when there is disruption of the muscle fibers and the sheath with hematoma formation. Surgery is usually necessary in these cases.

Early treatment is necessary to treat the primary muscle injury and prevent excessive fibrous tissue formation during the healing phase. Ice, rest, and gentle massage are used to reduce the amount of local swelling. As recovery continues, deep friction massage and stretching may begin after resolution of acute inflammation. Therapeutic laser and therapeutic ultrasound may be useful in the early phases of treatment. Activity and exercise are increased depending on the severity of injury and the response to treatment. It is important to progress the intensity of the program rather slowly to avoid reinjury and setbacks. Muscles sustaining injury and undergoing healing may be more susceptible to reinjury. Therefore, it is wise to be vigilant about rehabilitation and resume training slowly, with frequent monitoring of the patient.

Fibrotic Myopathy

Fibrotic myopathy is the pathologic replacement of muscle fibers with dense connective tissue and is a much more serious condition to treat. There are fibrous bands within the muscle, leading to lameness and restricted ROM. The semitendinosus, semimembranosus, biceps femoris, gracilis, and triceps muscles are most commonly affected. Studies of fibrotic myopathy have reported that up to 61% of cases occur bilaterally.[31] German shepherd dogs, Doberman pinschers, and racing greyhounds are most frequently affected, although other breeds may also be affected. There is usually some history of muscle trauma, especially repetitive trauma in active dogs. There may also be severe trauma to the muscle as a result of sudden stops.

There may be lameness of the affected limb, decreased ROM, the presence of fibrous bands on palpation, and, in the case of fibrotic myopathy of the gracilis or hamstring muscles, a characteristic jerking-type gait during the swing phase with external rotation of the hock and internal rotation of the stifle.

As with many athletic injuries, the best treatment of fibrotic myopathy is prevention. Proper warmup and cooldown with each exercise or competition session are recommended. Dogs must be evaluated by their owners for any pain on palpation, swelling, or lameness. If problems are found, professional attention should be sought. If a muscle injury is detected in the acute phase, rest and ice are implemented. Later stages are treated with appropriate stretching and strengthening.

After chronic fibrotic myopathy has occurred, the authors adopt an aggressive approach to management, including surgical removal of all fibrous bands followed by in-house rehabilitation for 1 month and outpatient and home therapy for 4 to 6 months. Historically, the reported outcome for surgical treatment of fibrotic myopathy has been poor.[31,32] However, if the fibrotic bands are aggressively resected and intense rehabilitation is used to prevent recurrence, the animal can return to acceptable function, although generally at a lower level.

After surgery, the authors hospitalize the patient for 4 weeks to maintain complete control over the rehabilitation program. If progress is acceptable, a transition to outpatient therapy may begin during weeks 4 to 8, 2 to 3 times per week, with a home exercise program every day between sessions. The home exercise program continues in the third month, with weekly rechecks. The home exercise program continues with monthly rechecks for a total of 6 months. If at any time there is evidence of recurrence, the patient is reevaluated and appropriate corrections are made.

In-house therapy begins while the patient is recovering from anesthesia, with cryotherapy and PROM. Cryotherapy is continued 3 to 4 times per day for 20 minutes until resolution of acute inflammation. Gentle PROM is continued 3 to 6 times per day for 20 repetitions during the entire time of hospitalization and during the home exercise program. Gentle massage to the area is also initiated. Gentle stretching along with the PROM begins within 2 to 3 days postoperatively and continues during the home exercise program and is especially important, not only in treatment but also as a monitoring tool to detect any worsening of the condition. Muscle-specific stretches with anatomic positioning of joints to achieve maximal stretch are used whenever possible. For example, maximum stretch of the hamstring muscles may be achieved by extending the stifle and slowly flexing the hip joint until mild discomfort is achieved and then holding for 15 seconds (**Fig. 5**). If there is pain or resistance with stretching, it may be beneficial to use a coaptation device to maintain the muscle in an elongated position for several hours daily. The authors use therapeutic ultrasound and therapeutic laser in an attempt to achieve healing as quickly as possible and maturation of any healing scar tissue while the animal is hospitalized and under their care. Weight shifting is initiated the day after surgery to encourage weight-bearing on the affected limb and contraction and relaxation of muscle tissue in the limb. Slow leash walks are also initiated as well as abduction and adduction exercises, such as lateral walking, especially if the gracilis or hamstring muscles are affected (**Fig. 6**). Cavaletti rails are instituted as soon as the patient is able in an attempt to have the patient have greater active ROM. Other therapeutic exercises that target increases in active ROM of specific affected joints are also incorporated. Underwater treadmill walking may begin during week 2 if appropriate progress is made. Strengthening and swimming exercises may begin in week 3 or 4. Finally, the dog begins to gradually return to speed activities during weeks 8 to 12, with a goal of complete return by 16 to 20 weeks.

Iliopsoas Muscle Conditions

Iliopsoas muscle conditions are an increasingly recognized condition in dogs with pain near the coxofemoral joint that is not related to OA. Patients may have a mild lameness. During examination, patients may not have pain with simple flexion and

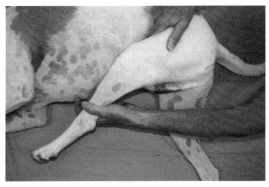

Fig. 5. Hamstring stretch. Note the hip is flexed, and the stifle is slowly extended until initial discomfort is achieved. The stretch is held for 15 to 60 seconds.

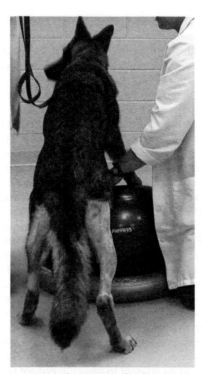

Fig. 6. Lateral motion is encouraged after surgery for fibrotic myopathy of the gracillis muscle by having the dog move around an inflatable donut.

extension of the hip joint, but when the hip is extended with simultaneous internal or external rotation of the hip, or if pressure is applied to the muscle or the insertion of the iliopsoas tendon on the lesser trochanter, dogs are often in extreme pain.[33,34] It is important to note the anatomy of the region.[34] The lesser trochanter is on the medial side of the femur, located on the caudal portion of the bone caudal to the pectineus muscle. The femoral nerve is in close association with the iliopsoas muscle and may be compressed if there is muscle swelling. Pain is also sometimes elicited on palpation of the iliacus muscle origin on the medial aspect of the body of the ilium. In cases of acute muscle damage, diagnostic ultrasound may indicate hemorrhage and fibrosis. Most cases of iliopsoas pain and discomfort are secondary to an underlying problem, such as OA of the hip or stifle joint. With reduced active extension of these joints and decreased propulsion, the iliopsoas muscle may undergo adaptive shortening and, when stretched to a normal degree, may be uncomfortable. Nevertheless, it is important to treat all conditions that may hinder return to function. Most of the secondary cases of iliopsoas discomfort may be treated with a program of heating and targeted stretching, along with massage. Further diagnostic evaluation includes ultrasound and MRI evaluation. These techniques are also useful to help determine if the condition is acute with edema and hematoma formation or chronic with fibrosis.

Cases with pathologic abnormality of the iliopsoas muscle may be treated conservatively with strict rest for 10 to 12 weeks, along with initial cryotherapy, gentle stretching and cross-frictional massage, and NSAIDs for 1 week.[33] Treatments should be comfortable for the patient and not cause excessive pain. Two or 3 treatments of low energy extracorporeal shock-wave administered every other week may be beneficial for healing and pain control. Therapeutic ultrasound and therapeutic laser 2 or 3 times weekly may also help the recovery. PRP injections administered early in the course of the condition may speed the reparative process because of the many growth factors provided to the healing tissues.[34] In many mild cases, conservative treatment is effective. In more severe cases, the tendon of insertion may be transected and pain relief is often dramatic.

Limber Tail

Limber tail is a condition typically seen in hunting dogs that swim in cold water or ride in the back of a truck in cold, damp weather conditions.[35] Dogs may be in pain when the condition first begins. The affected region of the tail is carried in a drooped position and they cannot raise the tail. There may be swelling just below the tail base. In general, dogs are relatively normal within a few days, but the condition may recur. Serum creatine kinase concentrations may be elevated and EMG abnormalities of the affected portions of the tail muscles may be noted. NSAIDs may be beneficial early in the disease process.

REHABILITATION OF TENDON AND LIGAMENT CONDITIONS

A variety of tendon and ligament injuries occur in small animal practice. With the popularity of canine sporting events, increasing attention is being paid to these structures. Rehabilitation of tendon and ligament conditions using basic biology of healing principles coupled with the biomechanical stresses placed on healing tissues by patients is emphasized following injury and surgical repair.

Basic Biology of Tendon and Ligament Rehabilitation

It is well-established that prolonged immobilization following repair results in decreased tensile strength of healing tendons and ligaments.[36] The sutured medial collateral ligament of dogs immobilized for 3 weeks followed by active motion had valgus-varus stifle joint laxity of 150% and ultimate ligament strength of 92% compared with intact controls.[37] Prolonging the period of immobilization to 6 weeks resulted in laxity of 300% and only 14% of ultimate strength compared with intact control dogs. Therefore, it seems that immobilization for 3 to 4 weeks allows sufficient strength to allow protected active motion. By 6 weeks, tendons have approximately 50% of tensile strength (it is estimated that 25%–33% of strength is needed to withstand physiologic muscle contractions).

Early passive motion increases tensile strength and ultimate load of healing tissues 2 to 3 times more than if the tissues are immobilized.[38] In addition, adhesions are reduced with early motion. On the other hand, dogs that are too active or owners that do not comply with postoperative exercise restrictions may place too much stress on healing tissues, resulting in treatment failure. Excessive excursions of joints with gap formation at the repair site are detrimental to healing. It is important to protect the repair, yet allow some motion of tissues and joints.[39]

Increasing the rate of passive motion may have beneficial effects. For example, passive motion of healing canine digital flexor tendons at 12 cycles per minute for 5 minutes daily had similar gliding function with significantly greater tensile properties than 1 cycle per minute for 60 minutes.[40]

The basic principles of rehabilitation following tendon injury should be considered:

- Maintain ROM to combat the deleterious effects of immobilization
- Avoid excessive excursions
- Protect the damaged tendon from adverse stress

- Apply low cyclic loads to promote ligament/tendon matrix formation and enhance remodeling
- Progressively increase the frequency and magnitude of loading to the healing ligament/tendon

NSAIDs should be used judiciously after tendon and ligament surgery because these drugs can have a negative effect on tendon healing in the early proliferative phase. They may be beneficial in the remodeling phase, however, if low-grade inflammation is present. Fluoroquinolone antibiotics should be avoided because of negative effects on fibroblast metabolism, especially in tendons and ligaments.[41] Their use should be reserved for life-threatening infections when tendon or ligament injury is present.

Sprains and Strains

Strains occur relatively commonly, but they are frequently undiagnosed or underdiagnosed. Dogs with mild injuries may be rested and treated conservatively. The other extreme is carpal hyperextension syndrome, a serious sprain involving the carpal ligaments and palmar fibrocartilage that generally requires fusion of the all or some of the carpal joints.

Strains of the biceps and supraspinatus muscles may occur, especially in dogs that frequently jump or are trained in muddy conditions. Infraspinatus muscle contracture is a well-recognized condition. Tendinopathies, such as those involving the Achilles tendon, are primarily degenerative conditions; there is usually an absence of inflammatory cells in or around the lesion.

Although some injuries are unavoidable, prevention of injuries is preferable to having a major injury. The optimal prevention program involves proper selection of a dog for a particular event, initiating training at the proper age, proper warm-up and cool-down periods (including stretching), having an appropriate conditioning and training program, educating owners regarding evaluation of their dog after each workout, and regular veterinary evaluations to be certain that overuse injuries are not occurring.

Tendon Lacerations

Most severe tendon injuries are generally the result of trauma and should be surgically repaired as soon as possible. Digital flexor or extensor tendon lacerations are frequently repaired by suturing the tendon ends together. Open wounds should be appropriately managed by debriding tissue and managing contamination to prevent infection. Repair should be initiated when the wound is deemed healthy for surgery. Appropriate suture and suture patterns should be applied to reappose tendon or ligament ends. The 3-loop pulley and double-locking loop suture patterns are used most frequently.

The greatest risk of failure following flexor tendon transection and repair is in the early period after repair. The most common risk factors associated with failure are the development of repair site elongation and rupture and the formation of adhesions within the digital sheath.[42] These complications are due primarily to the failure of the repair site to accrue strength within the first few weeks after suture repair, exacerbated by a posttraumatic increase in gliding resistance.

The use of growth factors may significantly speed the healing process and strength gain of healing tissues, especially when incorporated in a carrier or delivery system.[42] Bioengineered porcine small-intestinal submucosa (SIS) may provide support to the area of repair by placing it around the repaired area. Collagen deposition, neovascularization, and tensile strength may be enhanced with SIS.[43] Hyaluronic acid gel placed around healing tendons should also be considered. A significantly faster increase in breaking strength was found in hyaluronic acid gel-treated compared with saline-treated tendons in one study, which coincided with a significantly accelerated tissue repair response after injury. Improved gliding may also be noted.[44]

NSAIDs should be used judiciously after tendon and ligament surgery. Studies have indicated that these drugs can have a negative effect on tendon healing in the early proliferative phase, but might be beneficial in the remodeling phase when inflammation might impede healing. Fluoroquinolone antibiotics should be avoided after tendon surgery because of their negative effects on fibroblast metabolism.[41]

Too much activity after surgery frequently results in failure of the repair and a "dropped toe," which may lead to reluctance on the part of the veterinarian to repair the next case. Therefore, it is critical that patients (and owners) are compliant with postoperative restrictions. Healing of tendon injuries occurs slowly, and it is important to maintain adequate postoperative immobilization with splints, casts, or other external coaptation devices. Healing tendons have 56% tensile strength at 6 weeks and 79% tensile strength at 1 year.[36] Healing and recovery rates vary with age, severity of injury, and specific tissue damage.

Unfortunately, poor healing and even weakening of healing tissues may occur if there is no stress applied to the repaired tendons.[45] In fact, wound healing strength actually begins to decline if the limb is immobilized longer than 4 weeks. There is a fine balance between excessive loading and too much protection of the tissues to maximize healing and attaining strength. The therapist must initiate a rehabilitation program of controlled, gradual increases in loading and stress to tissues. The process may be long (and expensive), but excellent results may be expected in most cases.

Postsurgically, the surgical limb is immobilized for a period of time after surgery to allow initial healing and to prevent catastrophic failure and gap formation. Whenever possible, tension is reduced on the healing tissue by proper positioning before applying external coaptation. For example, the carpus is placed in a slightly flexed position to decrease tension on a sutured superficial digital flexor tendon. Three to 4 weeks of immobilization are generally adequate for most repairs. It is important to realize that stress on a healing tendon repair may result from muscle-tendon tension as a result of muscle contraction and weight-bearing forces. Muscle contraction forces are not completely eliminated, so there will be some physiologic stress to the tissues. However, the tendon must be protected from catastrophic weight-bearing forces. A circular external fixator ring or walking ring may be applied in conjunction

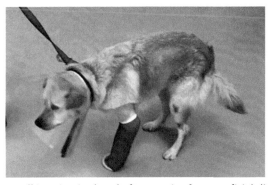

Fig. 7. A cast with a walking ring is placed after repair of a superficial digital flexor tendon repair.

with an external coaptation device so that the ring bears the forces of weight-bearing, relieving stress on the repair. The walking ring allows transfer of weight-bearing forces from the ground to proximal of the repair, bypassing the repair. As healing progresses, the walking ring is advanced proximally to allow shared weight-bearing with the foot, and eventually the walking ring is removed. The authors have found that a circular-shaped walking ring formed from aluminum splint rod or a circular external fixator ring with the circle placed flat on the ground works best and results in the most normal weight-bearing of the patient (**Fig. 7**).

Postoperative rehabilitation begins 3 to 4 days after repair. It is important to combine scientific knowledge with clinical common sense. The goal is to apply controlled tension and motion to prevent adhesions and improve healing, without damaging the repair. To avoid contracture of tissues, the digits should be gradually extended (for flexor tendon injuries) to apply controlled stress on the repair for 10 repetitions per day, such that the tendon is gliding only 1 to 2 mm. This movement will help to prevent adhesions while avoiding excessive gap formation of the repair. Depending on the quality of the tissues and strength of the repair, slight weight-bearing is allowed on the limb 3 or 4 weeks postoperatively by raising the walking ring to allow toe-touching. Dogs may be leash-walked 10 to 15 minutes, 3 to 4 times daily. Running, jumping, and playing are prohibited. The ring is raised every 7 to 10 days until the foot is completely weight-bearing, usually by 6 to 8 weeks postoperatively. For the next 6 to 8 weeks, a protective device is worn on the limb, such as a commercial or custom-made splint or brace, between home exercise sessions

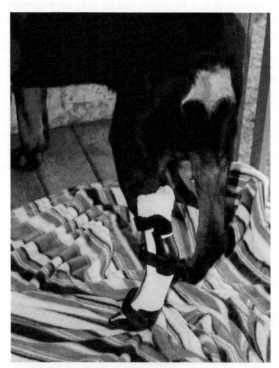

Fig. 8. A commercial splint is applied to help protect a tendon repair from catastrophic failure in the late recovery phase following surgery. The splint may be removed when the dog is under strict control, but is replaced when not attended.

(**Fig. 8**). During this time, dog may be walked without any coaptation for 5 minutes, 3 to 5 times daily, increasing the walks by 5 minutes per week. Slow trotting may begin on the limb 10 weeks postoperatively, beginning with 1 to 2 minutes per session, and increasing the length of time by 10 to 15% per week. The entire healing and rehabilitation period may be 4 to 6 months depending on the severity of injury, condition of the dog, and response to therapy. If lameness or tendon injury occurs at any point, the rehabilitation intensity must be reduced until the condition resolves.

Calcaneal Tendon

Although the common calcaneal tendon is indeed a tendon, there are special considerations in treatment and rehabilitation. The tendon is essential to normal weight-bearing and function of the pelvic limb. Although primary laceration and disruption occur, the tendon is frequently afflicted with a degenerative condition, usually with an absence of inflammatory cells in or around the lesion. Although some surgeons recommend pantarsal arthrodesis of the hock to prevent excessive hock flexion during weight-bearing (dropped hock), tarsal motion is vital to functions, such as stepping over obstacles, climbing stairs, sitting, and so on. Surgical fusion of the hock requires the stifle and hip joints to compensate for the loss of hock function, potentially exacerbating pre-existing conditions of these joints. Therefore, whenever possible and feasible, repair of the tendon is recommended. The process is lengthy and costly,

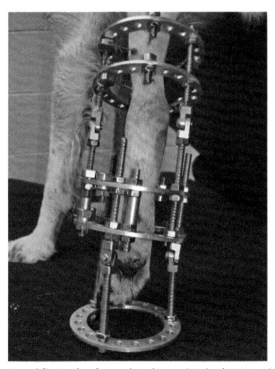

Fig. 9. A circular external fixator has been placed to maintain the tarsus in an extended position. A walking ring has been placed at the bottom of the fixator to prevent weight-bearing on the foot in the very early postoperative period following repair of a common calcaneal tendon injury.

but very good results may be expected. The principles of tendon rehabilitation previously outlined are followed, with some exceptions.

Following repair of the common calcaneal tendon of large dogs, the tarsus should be rigidly immobilized. One option is a transarticular external skeletal fixator with a walking ring placed and the tarsus maintained in an extended position to reduce resting stress on the healing tendon (**Fig. 9**). Recent research has indicated that muscle stress on the tendon is similar during weight-bearing, regardless of tarsal immobilization.[46] Placement of a walking ring may reduce stress on the tendon by transferring weight-bearing forces from the ground to proximal to the repair, bypassing the repair. Beginning on day 3 postoperatively, the digits are flexed and extended 10 times per day, with only 1 to 2 mm of excursion in the first 2 weeks. Excursions may be slowly increased beginning 3 weeks after repair. Also at 3 weeks, additional flexion (3–5°) may be applied to the tarsus so that stress is gradually introduced to healing tissue. As healing progresses, the walking ring is advanced proximally to allow shared weight-bearing with the foot, and eventually the walking ring is removed. Four weeks after repair, the ring is raised to barely allow some toe-touching. The ring is raised every 7 to 10 days, until the foot is completely weight-bearing, generally by 8 weeks after surgery. At the same time, the hock is positioned with more flexion until a normal standing position is achieved. Whenever adjustments are made, it is advisable to put the hock and other joints through ROM exercises. It is important to keep the coaptation device in place between adjustments to prevent catastrophic failure of the repair. During the transition to complete weight-bearing on the foot, the dog is initially allowed 3 to 5 minutes of slow leash walking 3 to 4 times per day, increasing 10% to 15% per week. If possible, transition to increased motion of the joint may be instituted 8 to 10 weeks after surgery using a hinge with the ability to "lock out" excessive flexion.

After 12 to 16 weeks, the external fixator or other coaptation device may be removed. The repair is protected with a walking splint/boot when the dog is not under direct control to prevent catastrophic failure. The dog may be walked without any coaptation for 5 minutes, 3 to 5 times daily, increasing the walks by 5 minutes per week. Slow trotting may begin on the limb 14 to 16 weeks postoperatively, beginning with 1 to 2 minutes per session, and increasing the length of time by 10% to 15% per week. The entire healing and rehabilitation period may be 5 to 8 months depending on the severity of injury, condition of the dog, and response to therapy. If lameness or tendon injury occurs at any point, the rehabilitation intensity must be reduced until the condition resolves.

Controlled introduction of angular joint motion and weight-bearing stress over a period of time is critical. The entire process may take weeks to months, but patience and proper application of forces within the strength of healing tissues can give excellent results.

Modalities That May Be Useful in Tendon and Ligament Healing

A variety of modalities may be beneficial in tendon and ligament healing (**Table 1**). Therapeutic laser, therapeutic ultrasound, extracorporeal shock-wave, therapeutic exercises, and biologic modalities are described and may have use in promoting healing of tendons and ligaments.

Therapeutic Laser in Tendon and Ligament Healing

Therapeutic laser has been recommended for various tendon conditions, but the clinical efficacy remains controversial. Therapeutic laser is increasingly used in rehabilitative applications to decrease pain, reduce inflammatory processes, and promote tissue healing in people with Achilles tendon problems. One study evaluated

Table 1
Physical rehabilitation modalities potentially useful in the treatment of tendon and ligament injuries, and their proposed mechanism of action

Treatment	Proposed Mechanism of Action
Decreased activity	Prevention of injury or re-injury
Cryotherapy	Reduction of inflammation and cell metabolism
Thermotherapy	Improve blood flow, nutrient delivery, and cell metabolism
Physical rehabilitation	Stimulate cell activity, blood flow, and remodeling of tissues
Eccentric exercise	Stimulate cell activity and remodeling of cell matrix
NMES	Pain control, stimulate cell activity and blood flow
Therapeutic laser	Increase cell metabolism, pain control
Therapeutic ultrasound	Stimulate cell metabolism and blood flow, heat tissues
Extracorporeal shock-wave treatment	Stimulate cell metabolism, blood flow, neovascularization, growth factor release and pain relief
NSAIDs	Reduce inflammation (may also inhibit wound healing if used early)
Glycosaminoglycans	Reduce metalloproteinase activity, stimulate production of extracellular matrix
PRP	Provide multiple growth factors, including TGF-β, platelet-derived growth factor, promoting tissue repair
Stem cell therapy	Reduce inflammation, aid in tissue repair and remodeling

therapeutic laser in people with bilateral Achilles tendinitis.[47] Therapeutic laser (904 nm, 5.4 J per point, 20 mW/cm^2) or placebo was randomly applied to either Achilles tendon in people. Prostaglandin E_2 was reduced, and pain pressure threshold values increased 75 to 105 minutes after laser treatment.

Therapeutic laser increased cell proliferation, type I collagen mRNA, and gene expression of porcine Achilles tendon fibroblasts in another study.[48] Laser therapy was also effective in improving collagen fiber organization of the calcanean tendon after undergoing a partial lesion.[49]

A review and meta-analysis evaluated therapeutic laser for tendinopathies.[19] The results of 25 studies were conflicting. Roughly half of the studies suggested a positive effect, whereas the other half was inconclusive or had no effect. Overall, positive results were found in people with lateral epicondylitis and Achilles tendinopathy, with the results related to the dose of laser applied. Studies suggest that therapeutic laser was efficacious when doses of 1 to 8 J and power less than 100 mW/cm^2 were used for superficial tendons. For deeper tendons, such as the rotator cuff, power up to 600 mW/cm^2 and total dosages of 3 to 9 J have been recommended in people. These doses have not been evaluated in dogs for tendon and ligament conditions.

Therapeutic Ultrasound

Therapeutic ultrasound may be used for thermal and nonthermal effects. The thermal effects may result in decreased pain and muscle spasm, and increased collagen extensibility. The nonthermal or biologic effects include acceleration of the inflammatory phase of wound healing with a quicker entry into the proliferative phase of repair, stimulation of fibroblast proliferation, promotion of stronger and more elastic scar tissue as a result of increased collagen formation and changes in collagen fiber pattern, and changes in membrane permeability that may speed the healing process.[50]

Low-intensity pulsed ultrasound results in up-regulation of biglycan and collagen I gene expression. Ultrasound also results in faster healing rates in injured tendons and ligaments. However, the optimal time and duration of treatment have not yet been determined. One study suggested that pulsed ultrasound promoted restoration of mechanical strength and collagen alignment in healing tendons only when applied in the early healing stages.[51,52]

Extracorporeal Shockwave Treatment

Extracorporeal shock-wave treatment uses high-intensity acoustic waves with a rapidly rising pulse pressure to stimulate tissue healing. Extracorporeal shock-wave treatment has been used to treat tendinopathies with encouraging short-term results in people. One protocol studied in people with Achilles tendinopathy consisted of 4 sessions, at a 2- to 7-day interval.[53] Five hundred pulses were applied with energy of 0.08 and 0.40 mJ/mm^2. Satisfactory results were seen in 47.2% of cases at 2 months, 73.2% at medium-term follow-up, and 76% in the last evaluation. Others have reviewed the use of extracorporeal shockwave treatment for musculoskeletal conditions in people and animal models.[54]

Therapeutic Exercise

Studies in people indicate positive results from eccentric training in patients with tendon disorders. The reasons eccentric exercises are beneficial are not completely known. In one study, eccentric exercises to treat tendinopathy conservatively in people were equivalent to extracorporeal shock-wave therapy and were superior to conservative treatment.[55]

Other Treatments

Other treatments that have been recommended for tendon and ligament injuries include autogenous stem cell injection, PRP, prolotherapy, polysulfated glycosaminoglycans, and compounds containing glucosamine and chondroitin sulfate. In particular, the biologic treatments of PRP and stem cell therapy show great promise. These substances possess relatively large amounts of growth factors and other substances that may improve the speed and quality of repair. Additional research will help to further define the roles, efficacy, dosages, and frequency of treatment to achieve optimal healing.

Summary

Proper postoperative treatment and rehabilitation of tendon and ligament injuries are critical to success. After repair, the area should be immobilized for 3 to 4 weeks with the limb placed such that the affected tissues are in a shortened position. PROM exercises should be started early with tendon excursions of 1 to 2 mm. Weight-bearing stresses should gradually be increased, and sudden bursts of exercise that could damage healing tissues should be avoided. Also, protection of the repair should be continued as weight-bearing stresses are increased on the tissues. The use of specific rehabilitation exercises and modalities to improve motion, limb use, and tissue healing should be considered.

OSTEOARTHRITIS

OA is a common problem, affecting up to 60% of dogs.[56] Patients with OA have restricted activity, limited ability to perform, muscle atrophy, pain and discomfort, decreased ROM, and decreased quality of life. As animals reduce their activity level, a vicious cycle of decreased flexibility, joint stiffness, and loss of strength occurs.

Traditional management of dogs with OA has included anti-inflammatory and anal-gesic drugs, changes in lifestyle, and surgical management. Advances in the manage-ment of human and canine OA have included physical modalities, such as thermal modalities, exercise, TENS, therapeutic ultrasound, therapeutic laser, and extracorpo-real shockwave treatment to reduce the severity of symptoms and reliance on medi-cations to control pain and discomfort; this article focuses on these other modalities. Caution should be used in the application of these modalities, and they should only be applied by those that are trained in their proper use.

Thermal Modalities

Heat and cold have been used to manage OA. Ice massage may be particularly useful for helping to improve function. Heat therapy may be useful to help improve flexibility and ROM in arthritic patients. Therapeutic ultrasound may have a positive effect on stiffness and pain through its thermal effects.

Therapeutic Exercises

Comprehensive studies of therapeutic exercises in dogs with OA have not been per-formed to date. However, anecdotal evidence suggests that low-impact therapeutic exercises in dogs, especially aquatic exercises, are effective in dogs, as they are in people. One study of swimming and clinical function of dogs with osteoarthritic hip joints suggested that twice weekly swimming for 8 weeks improved lameness, joint mobility, weight-bearing, pain on palpation, and overall score.[57] A recent study of peo-ple with knee OA randomized to aquatic or land-based exercises indicated that both water-based and land-based exercises reduced knee pain and increased knee func-tion in participants. Hydrotherapy was superior to land-based exercise in relieving pain before and after walking during the last follow-up.[58] Well-designed studies of exercise and OA in dogs are needed.

Transcutaneous Electrical Nerve Stimulation

TENS is a form of electrical stimulation (ES). A wide variety of ES and TENS units are available. Neuromuscular electrical stimulation provides several benefits including increasing muscle strength and joint ROM, decreasing edema and pain, and helping to improve function. Pulsed alternating current units are the most useful for increasing muscle strength and joint ROM, and decreasing edema and pain. The commonly used TENS refers only to a particular type of electrical stimulation that is applied for pain control, but is not used for muscle strengthening or other applications.

TENS is a relatively inexpensive, safe, noninvasive modality with few side effects that can be used to treat a variety of painful conditions. The clinical application of TENS involves the delivery of an electrical current to the skin by surface electrodes. Conventional TENS stimulators most commonly used in animals are high frequency (40–150 Hz, 50–100 μs pulse width, low to moderate intensity) because they are more comfortable and create less anxiety in small animal patients.

TENS provides analgesia by several potential mechanisms of action, including the "gate theory" of pain control. People describe a "pins-and-needle" sensation under the electrodes, resulting in paresthesia. Endogenous opiates may be released and result in pain relief by stimulating the descending pain-inhibiting pathway. Low-frequency TENS analgesia may be mediated by activation of serotonin and μ-opioid receptors, while conventional TENS activates δ-opioid receptors.

A meta-analysis concluded that TENS used for chronic knee OA in people resulted in relatively positive results.[59] Although there is evidence that TENS is effective in managing the pain of knee OA in people, it is less certain whether TENS treatment is effective in improving physical function. A recent study examined the effects of a single treatment with TENS on osteoarthritic pain in the stifle of dogs.[60] Although all dogs started with mild decreases in weight-bearing as assessed by force plate analysis of gait, dogs receiving a 30-minute TENS application had a significant increase in weight-bearing 30 minutes after treatment, and these differences persisted for 210 minutes after TENS application. The magnitude of increase was similar to that which is typically expected of NSAIDs. Although there are some disadvantages of TENS application, including the expertise necessary to use the equipment and the necessity of daily application, it may give added benefit to medications and may be used in patients who cannot tolerate certain medications.

Therapeutic Ultrasound

Therapeutic ultrasound has been suggested as being beneficial for patients with OA through its thermal and nonthermal biologic effects. Specific studies of arthritic dogs have not been performed, but there is some evidence that it may be useful in people with OA. A recent meta-analysis evaluated the use of therapeutic ultrasound in 5 small-sized trials with a total of 341 patients with knee OA.[61] Two evaluated pulsed ultrasound; 2 evaluated continuous, and one evaluated both pulsed and continuous ultrasound as the active treatment. For pain, there was an effect in favor of ultrasound therapy, which corresponded to a 12% improvement. There was also a favorable improvement in function with ultrasound treatment. The authors concluded that therapeutic ultrasound may be beneficial for patients with OA of the knee, justifying further appropriately designed trials of adequate power.

Therapeutic Laser

Therapeutic laser affects photochemical reactions in the cell (photobiomodulation). Many different types of laser are used for medical purposes. Therapeutic lasers used for rehabilitation techniques are thought to have positive effects on tissues, as compared with high-power surgical lasers that are designed for thermal destruction of tissues. Class IVa therapeutic lasers have intermediate power. Laser light is collimated, coherent, and monochromatic. These properties allow laser light to penetrate the skin surface without damage to the skin or heating effect.

Therapeutic laser has been used to treat OA. Although results from therapeutic laser treatment of pain have been controversial, 635-nm low-level laser therapy has been approved for human use by the US Food and Drug Administration for the management of chronic minor pain, as in OA and muscle spasms. Laser treatment was performed on human patients with OA of the knee in one study.[62] A pulsed infrared diode laser, 810-nm wavelength, was used once per day for 5 consecutive days, followed by a 2-day rest interval. The total number of applications was 12 sessions. There was significant improvement in pain relief and quality of life in 70% of patients. Although the authors of this study indicated that laser treatment was beneficial, there was not an untreated control group. Therefore, the results should be interpreted with caution. Another study of 90 patients with knee OA evaluated gallium arsenide laser therapy in combination with 30 minutes of exercise.[63] One group received 5 minutes of therapeutic laser, with 3 J delivered. Another group was treated for 3 minutes and received 2 J, while a third group received placebo laser and exercise. Patients received a total of 10 treatments and were studied for 14 weeks. Patients receiving laser treatment had significantly improved pain, function, and quality-of-life measures after treatment and had improved scores as compared with the placebo laser group.

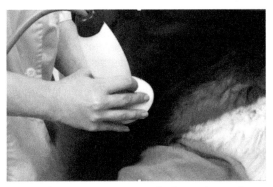

Fig. 10. Extracorporeal shock-wave treatment applied to a dog with OA of the elbow joint.

Extracorporeal Shockwave Therapy

Extracorporeal shockwaves are a focused pulse of high-pressure acoustic waves of various frequencies that travel through soft tissue to reach their target area. When the shockwave reaches a density interface (eg, ligament or bone), energy is released. The larger the change in impedance, the greater the energy released. It is this energy release that is thought to stimulate healing. When a shockwave travels through the target area, very high pressures build up for a very short period of time; energy is released, and the pressure returns to normal. Orthopedic applications for which shockwave therapy is useful in people include nonunion fractures, plantar fasciitis, lateral epicondylitis, Achilles and patella tendonitis, and, with limited experience, OA. Shockwave treatment has also been used in horses to treat suspensory ligament desmitis, tendinopathies, navicular disease, back pain, OA, and stress fractures. Although treatment of dogs with shockwave therapy is relatively new, tendonitis, desmitis, spondylosis, nonunion fractures, and OA have all been successfully treated (**Fig. 10**).

The clinical effects of shockwave treatment include reduced inflammation and swelling, short-term analgesic effect, improved vascularity and neovascularization, increased bone formation, realignment of tendon fibers, and enhanced wound healing. The mechanisms of action that that underlie the clinical effects are not clearly understood, but studies have indicated that there is an induction of cytokines, such as TGF-β_1, Substance P, and osteocalcin. In addition, there is induction of nitric oxide synthase and increased osteoblastic activity. There may also be stimulation of nociceptors that inhibit afferent pain signals.

The authors have completed a study evaluating the use of extracorporeal shockwave therapy for the treatment of OA in dogs.[64] In this study, dogs with moderate to severe OA of the hip or elbow that had obvious clinical signs of lameness and pain were treated. Patients receiving shock-wave treatment demonstrated significant increases in weight-bearing and comfortable joint ROM, similar to what is typically expected with the use of NSAIDs. A larger follow-up study of only dogs with elbow OA had similar positive findings.[65] In fact, the improvement in peak vertical forces in dogs was nearly identical to the previous study. In addition, braking forces on the treated limbs were increased compared with untreated controls. In both studies, sham-treated dogs were offered treatment after the study was completed. These dogs that had no significant improvement with sham treatment had increased weight-bearing, similar to dogs in the treated group. Further study of shock-wave treatment is warranted to determine more optimal treatment protocols, including the frequency of treatment, energy level, and the number of impulses per treatment.

Miscellaneous Treatments

Prolotherapy may be beneficial in the management of OA. Prolotherapy typically involves injection of a dextrose solution into an arthritic joint. Some benefits have been reported in people. Botulinum toxin has also shown promise when injected intra-articularly in arthritic patients, including dogs. Several herbal treatments have been reported for treating OA. Many of these have been studied and have a physiologic basis, such as green tea, cat's claw, and Boswellia.

Biological therapies include interleukin receptor antagonist protein (IRAP), PRP, and stem cell therapy. IRAP may be beneficial by neutralizing one of the primary inflammatory mediator responsible for OA, interleukin-1. PRP is made from the patient's own blood and may be harvested in a relatively short period of time. It is a rich source of growth factors and helps to normalize the anabolic/catabolic balance in arthritic joints. Initial results have been promising. Stem cell therapy may be performed using mesenchymal stromal fraction stem cell therapy or cultured mesenchymal cells from the bone marrow. Although positive results have been reported, the treatments are relatively expensive.

Summary

Management of the arthritic patient involves several modalities and must be tailored to each patient. Weight control, physical rehabilitation, and medication are the main components for OA management. A variety of emerging physical modalities are available for the treatment of canine OA. Cooperation among the veterinarian, therapist, veterinary technician, and owner are vital to carry out an appropriate management program.

REFERENCES

1. Millis D, Levine D. Canine rehabilitation and physical therapy. 2nd edition. Philadelphia: Elsevier; 2014.
2. Davidson JR, Kerwin SC, Millis DL. Rehabilitation for the orthopedic patient. Vet Clin North Am Small Anim Pract 2005;35(6):1357–88.
3. Beale BS, Cole G. Minimally invasive osteosynthesis technique for articular fractures. Vet Clin North Am Small Anim Pract 2012;42:1051–68.
4. Hudson CC, Pozzi A. Minimally invasive repair of central tarsal bone luxation in a dog. Vet Comp Orthop Traumatol 2012;25:79–82.
5. Parker RB. Physeal Injuries. In: Bloomberg MS, Dee JF, Taylor RA, editors. Canine sports medicine and surgery. Philadelphia: Saunders; 1998. p. 223–34.
6. Piermattei DL, Flo GL, DeCamp CE. Brinker, Piermattei, and Flo's handbook of small animal orthopedics and fracture repair. 4th edition. St Louis (MO): Elsevier Saunders; 2006.
7. Davis S, Worth AJ. Successful return to work after surgical repair of fracture of the medial condyle of the distal femur in two working farm dogs. N Z Vet J 2009; 57(1):58–62.
8. Moores AP, Sutton A. Management of quadriceps contracture in a dog using a static flexion apparatus and physiotherapy. J Small Anim Pract 2009;50(5): 251–4.
9. Taylor J, Tangner CH. Acquired muscle contractures in the dog and cat. A review of the literature and case report. Vet Comp Orthop Traumatol 2007;20: 79–85.
10. Farrell M, Trevail T, Marshall W, et al. Computed tomographic documentation of the natural progression of humeral intracondylar fissure in a cocker spaniel. Vet Surg 2011;40(8):966–71.

11. Robin D, Marcellin-Little DJ. Incomplete ossification of the humeral condyle in two Labrador retrievers. J Small Anim Pract 2001;42(5):231–4.
12. Morgan OD, Reetz JA, Brown DC, et al. Complication rate, outcome, and risk factors associated with surgical repair of fractures of the lateral aspect of the humeral condyle in dogs. Vet Comp Orthop Traumatol 2008;21(5):400–5.
13. Nortje J, Bruce WJ, Worth AJ. Surgical repair of humeral condylar fractures in New Zealand working farm dogs – long term outcome and owner satisfaction. N Z Vet J 2014;7:1–17.
14. Anderson TJ, Carmichael S, Miller A. Intercondylar humeral fracture in the dog: a review of 20 cases. J Small Anim Pract 1990;31:437–42.
15. Denny HR. Condylar fractures of the humerus in the dog – a review of 133 cases. J Small Anim Pract 1983;24:185–97.
16. Vannini R, Smeak DD, Olmstead ML. Evaluation of surgical repair of 135 distal humeral fractures in dogs and cats. J Am Anim Hosp Assoc 1988;24:537–45.
17. McKee WM, Macias C, Innes JF. Bilateral fixation of Y-T humeral condyle fractures via medial and lateral approaches in 29 dogs. J Small Anim Pract 2005; 46:217–26.
18. Gordon WJ, Besançon MF, Conzemius MG, et al. Frequency of post-traumatic osteoarthritis in dogs after repair of a humeral condylar fracture. Vet Comp Orthop Traumatol 2003;16:1–5.
19. Tumilty S, Munn J, McDonough S, et al. Low level laser treatment of tendinopathy: a systematic review with meta- analysis. Photomed Laser Surg 2010;28:3–16.
20. Wernham BG, Jerram RM, Warman CG. Bicipital tenosynovitis in dogs. Compend Contin Educ Vet 2008;30(10):537–52.
21. Stobie D, Wallace LJ, Lipowitz AJ, et al. Chronic bicipital tenosynovitis in dogs: 29 cases (1985-1992). J Am Vet Med Assoc 1996;207:201–7.
22. Venzin C, Ohlerth S, Koch D, et al. Extracorporeal shockwave therapy in a dog with chronic bicipital tenosynovitis. Schweiz Arch Tierheilkd 2004;146:136–41.
23. Laitinen OM, Flo GL. Mineralization of the supraspinatus tendon in dogs: a long-term follow-up. J Am Anim Hosp Assoc 2000;36(3):262–7.
24. Petit GD. Infraspinatus muscle contracture in dogs. Mod Vet Pract 1980;61:451–2.
25. Devor M, Sorby R. Fibrotic contracture of the canine infraspinatus muscle: pathophysiology and prevention by early surgical intervention. Vet Comp Orthop Traumatol 2006;19:117–21.
26. Dillon EA, Anderson LJ, Jones BR. Infraspinatus muscle contracture in a working dog. NZ Vet J 1989;37:32–4.
27. Carberry CA, Gilmore DR. Infraspinatus muscle contracture associated with trauma in a dog. J Am Vet Med Assoc 1986;188:533–4.
28. Cook JL, Renfro DC, Tomlinson JL, et al. Measurement of angles of abduction for diagnosis of shoulder instability in dogs using goniometry and digital image analysis. Vet Surg 2005;34:463–8.
29. Davidson JR, Kerwin SC. Common orthopedic conditions and their physical rehabilitation. In: Millis DL, Levine D, editors. Canine rehabilitation and physical therapy. 2nd edition. Philadelphia: Elsevier; 2014. p. 543–81.
30. Cook JL, Tomlinson JL, Fox DB, et al. Treatment of dogs diagnosed with medial shoulder instability using radiofrequency-induced thermal capsulorrhaphy. Vet Surg 2005;34:469–75.
31. Steiss JE. Muscle disorders and rehabilitation in canine athletes. Vet Clin North Am Small Anim Pract 2002;32:267–85.
32. Lewis DD, Shelton GD, Piras A, et al. Gracilis or semitendinosus myopathy in 18 dogs. J Am Anim Hosp Assoc 1997;33:177–88.

33. Breur GJ, Blevins WE. Traumatic injury of the iliopsoas muscle in three dogs. *J Am Vet Med Assoc* 1997;210:1631–4.
34. Cabon Q, Bolliger C. Iliopsoas muscle injury in dogs. Compendium: continuing education for veterinarians. 2013. p. E1–7. Available at: Vetlearn.com.
35. Steiss J, Braund K, Wright J, et al. Coccygeal muscle injury in English pointers (Limber tail). J Vet Intern Med 1999;13:540–8.
36. Montgomery RD. Healing of muscle, ligaments, and tendons. Semin Vet Med Surg (Small Anim) 1989;4:304–11.
37. Woo SL, Inoue M, McGurk-Burleson E, Gomez MA. Treatment of the medial collateral ligament injury. II: structure and function of canine knees in response to differing treatment regimens. Am J Sports Med 1987;15(1):22–9.
38. Gelberman RH, Woo SLY, Lothringer K. Effects of early intermittent passive immobilization on healing canine flexor tendons. J Hand Surg 1982;7A:170–5.
39. Gelberman RH, Boyer MI, Brodt MB, et al. The effect of gap formation at the repair site on the strength and excursion of intrasynovial flexor tendons - an experimental study on the early stages of tendon-healing in dogs. J Bone Joint Surg Am 1999;81A:975–82.
40. Takai S, Woo SLYL, Horibe S, et al. The effects of frequency and duration of controlled passive mobilization on tendon healing. J Orthop Res 1991;9:705–13.
41. Williams RJ, Attia E, Wickiewicz TL, et al. The effect of ciprofloxacin on tendon, paratenon, and capsular fibroblast metabolism. Am J Sports Med 2000;28:364–9.
42. Thomopoulos S. Research trends for flexor tendon repair. In: Merolli A, Joyce TJ, editors. Biomaterials in hand surgery. Springer-Verlag Italia; 2009. p. 107–25.
43. Badylak SF, Tullius R, Kokini K, et al. The use of xenogeneic small intestinal sub-mucosa as a biomaterial for Achilles tendon repair in a dog model. J Biomed Mater Res 1995;29:977–85.
44. Amiel D, Ishizue K, Billings E Jr, et al. Hyaluronan in flexor tendon repair. J Hand Surg Am 1989;14:837–43.
45. Thomopoulos S, Zampiakis E, Das R, et al. The effect of muscle loading on flexor tendon-to-bone healing in a canine model. J Orthop Res 2008;26:1611–7.
46. Lister SA, Renberg WC, Roush JK. Efficacy of immobilization of the tarsal joint to alleviate strain on the common calcaneal tendon in dogs. Am J Vet Res 2009;70:134–40.
47. Bjordal JM, Lopes-Martins RAB, Iversen VV. A randomised, placebo controlled trial of low level laser therapy for activated Achilles tendinitis with microdialysis measurement of peritendinous prostaglandin E2 concentrations. Br J Sports Med 2006;40:76–80.
48. Chen CH, Tsai JL, Wang YH, et al. Low-level laser irradiation promotes cell pro-liferation and mRNA expression of type I collagen and decorin in porcine Achilles tendon fibroblasts in vitro. J Orthop Res 2009;27:646–50.
49. Oliveira FS, Pinfildi CE, Parizoto NA, et al. Effect of low level laser therapy (830 nm) with different therapy regimens on the process of tissue repair in partial lesion calcaneous tendon. Lasers Surg Med 2009;41:272–6.
50. Tsai WC, Tang SFT, Liang FC. Effect of therapeutic ultrasound on tendons. Am J Phys Med Rehabil 2011;90:1068–73.
51. Fu S-C, Shum W-T, Hung L-K, et al. Low-intensity pulsed ultrasound on tendon healing. A study of the effect of treatment duration and treatment initiation. Am J Sports Med 2008;36:1742–9.
52. Saini NS, Roy KS, Bansal PS, et al. A preliminary study of the effect of ultrasound therapy on the healing of surgically severed Achilles tendons in five dogs. J Vet Med 2002;49:321–8.

53. Vulpiani MC, Trischitta D, Trovato P, et al. Extracorporeal shockwave therapy (ESWT) in Achilles tendinopathy. A long-term follow-up observational study. J Sports Med Phys Fitness 2009;49(2):171–6.
54. Wang C-J. Extracorporeal shockwave therapy in musculoskeletal disorders. J Orthop Surg Res 2012;7:1–8.
55. Rompe JD, Nafe B, Furia JP, et al. Eccentric loading, shock-wave treatment, or a wait-and-see policy for tendiopathy of the main body of tendo achillis. A randomized controlled trial. Am J Sports Med 2007;35(3):374–83.
56. Millis DL, Tichenor M, Hecht S. Prevalence of osteoarthritis in dogs undergoing routine dental prophylaxis. Proc World Small Animal Veterinary Association Meeting, Cape Town, S. Africa 2014.
57. Nganvongpanit K, Tanvisut S, Yano T, et al. Effect of swimming on clinical functional parameters and serum biomarkers in healthy and osteoarthritic dogs. ISRN Vet Sci 2014;459809. http://dx.doi.org/10.1155/2014/459809 eCollection.
58. Silva LE, Valim V, Pessanha AP, et al. Hydrotherapy versus conventional land-based exercise for the management of patients with osteoarthritis of the knee:a randomized clinical trial. Phys Ther 2008;88:12–21.
59. Osiri M, Welch V, Brosseau L, et al. Transcutaneous electrical nerve stimulation for knee osteoarthritis (review). Cochrane Database Syst Rev 2000;(4): CD002823. http://dx.doi.org/10.1002/14651858.CD002823.
60. Levine D, Johnston K, Price N, et al. The effect of transcutaneous electrical nerve stimulation (TENS) on dogs with osteoarthritis of the stifle. Proc of the 32nd Veterinary Orthopedic Society, Snowmass, CO, March 2005.
61. Rutjes AW, Nüesch E, Sterchi R, et al. Therapeutic ultrasound for osteoarthritis of the knee or hip. Cochrane Database Syst Rev 2010;(1):CD003132. http://dx.doi. org/10.1002/14651858.CD003132.pub2.
62. Djavid GE, Mortazavi SMJ, Basirnia A, et al. Low level laser therapy in musculoskeletal pain syndrome: pain relief and disability reduction. Lasers Surg Med 2003;152(Suppl 15):43.
63. Gur A, Cosut A, Sarac AJ, et al. Efficacy of different therapy regimens of low-power laser in painful osteoarthritis of the knee: a double-blind and randomized-controlled trial. Laser Surg Med 2003;33:330–8.
64. Francis DA, Millis DL, Evans M, et al. Clinical evaluation of extracorporeal shockwave therapy for management of canine osteoarthritis of the elbow and hip joint. Proceedings of the 31st Annual Conference Veterinary Orthopedic Society, Big Sky, Montana, February 22-27, 2004.
65. Millis DL, Drum M, Whitlock D. Complementary use of extracorporeal shockwave therapy on elbow osteoarthritis in dogs. Vet Comp Orthop Traumatol 2011;24(3):A1.

Rehabilitation and Physical Therapy for the Neurologic Veterinary Patient

Cory Sims, DVM, Rennie Waldron, DVM, Denis J. Marcellin-Little, DEDV*

KEYWORDS

- Physiotherapy • Pain management • Rehabilitation • Canine rehabilitation
- Neurology • Client education

KEY POINTS

- The etiology and location of neurologic injury or disease have a significant impact on the design of the rehabilitation program as well as patient prognosis.
- Rehabilitation patients should be clinically stable with all immediate critical care and surgical concerns addressed before starting a physiotherapy program.
- A variety of modalities are available to the rehabilitation therapist to aid in pain management and support tissue healing.
- The exercise therapy component of the physiotherapy program assists in restoring core strength and balance to facilitate transitional activities (sitting up, standing from sitting, turns, etc).
- Client education is a critical part of the rehabilitation of neurologic patients; clients often manage urination and assisted locomotion at home for extended periods of time.

INTRODUCTION

Neurologic patients are often severely compromised: They may be unable to move limbs, urinate, defecate, or transition from lateral recumbency into a sternal position. Rehabilitation therapy for the neurologic patient places a profound emphasis on nursing and supportive care to protect the patient from complications and preserve tissue strength and function during the recovery period. The role of the rehabilitation practitioner therefore often extends beyond the performance of physiotherapy treatments and includes nursing care, medical management of complications from recumbency, and client education and support. This role often lasts weeks to months. Key aspects of a comprehensive rehabilitation program include pain management, physiotherapy, careful patient monitoring, supportive care for the patient, and compassionate client communication.

Department of Clinical Sciences, College of Veterinary Medicine, North Carolina State University, NCSU CVM VHC #2563, 1052 William Moore Drive, Raleigh, NC 27607-4065, USA
* Corresponding author.
E-mail address: djmarcel@ncsu.edu

Vet Clin Small Anim 45 (2015) 123–143
http://dx.doi.org/10.1016/j.cvsm.2014.09.007
0195-5616/15/$ – see front matter © 2015 Elsevier Inc. All rights reserved.

INITIAL PATIENT ASSESSMENT

A thorough physical examination and diagnostic assessment is invaluable in developing an effective rehabilitation therapy program and setting realistic goals. The therapist should perform complete neurologic and orthopedic examinations before starting a rehabilitation therapy program. It is important to have an accurate record of the patient's condition at the start of therapy as well as documentation of specific problems because the clinical status of patients with neurologic disease or injury can change rapidly. For example, progressive myelomalacia can occur shortly after injury or surgery and progresses rapidly.[1] Furthermore, many neurologic patients present with 1 or more comorbidities that may or may not be related to their neurologic diagnosis. Careful note should be made of the presence of concurrent injuries from trauma, developmental or degenerative orthopedic diseases, obesity, endocrinopathies, respiratory or cardiac dysfunction, and the presence of infection in any major body system.

The assessment should seek to establish the neuroanatomic localization, level of pain, and any secondary complications that have developed subsequent to the primary injury or disease process. Accurate neurolocalization aids in the formulation of a differential diagnosis list and diagnostic plan and, once a primary diagnosis has already been determined, helps to establish the prognosis and prioritize tests and criteria that will be used to monitor a patient's progress. For instance, establishing and monitoring the presence or absence of deep pain perception is essential in determining the prognosis and following the progress of a patient with spinal cord injury. Localization of neurologic injury has been covered extensively elsewhere.[2]

Standardized scoring systems have been developed to objectively and thoroughly characterize the neurologic status of canine patients with acute spinal cord injury secondary to intervertebral disc herniations.[3] In daily practice, the use of an extensive scoring system is not essential, but it is important for clinicians to develop a consistent approach to describing and recording a patient's neurologic function and pain level so that the patient's response to treatment can be accurately assessed over time. Key indicators that should be recorded at the initial patient assessment and when periodic reassessment is performed are listed in **Box 1**. Baseline objective data such as thigh girth, goniometry, body weight, body condition scoring, stance analysis, force plate, and kinematic analysis (when available) may also be collected and recorded in the patient history during this initial assessment. For ambulatory patients, gait assessment is an invaluable tool for assessing the patient's current status and identifying specific problems to be addressed during the treatment sessions. Written descriptions of gait should be as detailed as possible with the therapist and assistant or assistants using a common set of descriptors consistently with each assessment. A video record of the patient's gait performing a standard set of tasks (walking overground, on a treadmill or underwater treadmill, trotting, circling, weaving, and stepping over obstacles) is often the most useful and accurate method for recording gait abnormalities.[4–6]

Whenever possible, the client should be interviewed to determine an accurate list of current medications or supplements, chronic or recurrent illnesses, and, most important, the level of performance to which the animal is expected or needed to return. A detailed description of the household or housing arrangement, including any unique features of the environment and information about the pet's daily routine, is helpful in determining the necessary skill set for a particular patient. This description should include types of flooring, presence of obstacles such as stairs or pet doors, feeding and exercise schedules and any other relevant details.

Box 1
Key indicators of patient status at initial assessment and reassessments

Neurolocalization

Intracranial

- Forebrain
- Brainstem
- Cerebellum

Spinal

- C1–C5
- C6–T2
- T3–L3
- L4–S3

Peripheral or neuromuscular

Combination

Functional Status

Ambulatory/nonambulatory

With or without motor function

   (Note limbs affected: tetra-, hemi-, para-, mono-)

With or without spinal reflexes

With or without postural reflexes

With or without nociception

With or without panniculus reflex

With or without bladder and bowel control

Pain score and location

0-*No resentment*; normal amount of movement

1-*Mild withdrawal*; mildly resists

2-*Moderate withdrawal*; body tenses; *may orient* to site; *may vocalize*

3-*Orients to site; forcible withdrawal* from manipulation; may vocalize or hiss or bite

4-*Tries to escape/prevent manipulation; bite/hiss*; marked guarding of area

Presence of comorbidities or complications

With or without obesity

With or without metabolic or endocrine dysfunction

With or without infectious disease

With or without orthopedic disease

With or without disruptions in skin integrity

PHYSIOTHERAPY FOR SPINAL CORD DISEASE

Spinal cord injury is the most common neurologic disease treated by most veterinary rehabilitation facilities. Early (ie, starting 1–2 weeks after injury) and intensive rehabilitation therapy for locomotion training after spinal cord trauma has been shown in experimental models and patients to accelerate the recovery of motor function and return to ambulation.[7–9] Trauma to the spinal cord occurs as compression, contusion, shearing, or distraction from external forces, such as acute intervertebral disc disease, fibrocartilaginous embolism, falls, and vehicular accidents. During the peracute stage, there is direct compression, hemorrhage, and tissue shearing, which cause immediate cell death via disruption of cell membranes and dissociation of intercellular connections. The immediate damage interferes with transmission of nerve signals past the point of injury and also triggers a cascade of retrograde signaling that identifies the location of the lesion and recruits inflammatory mediators and cells to the area. After the immediate injury, local swelling, ongoing hemorrhage, and persistent tissue debris in the spinal canal may continue to exert compressive forces on the spinal cord itself, resulting in ongoing neuronal stress. Even in the absence of persistent compression, ischemia, or decreased perfusion, local edema and secondary oxidative damage play a key role in the extent and severity of spinal cord injury. Of these, tissue perfusion may be the most responsive to physiotherapeutic intervention; thus, physiotherapy techniques and modalities that promote circulation are often central to the rehabilitation program for patients with spinal cord injury.

Patients with spinal cord injuries such as fibrocartilaginous embolism, spinal fracture/luxation, and Hansen type I intervertebral disc disease generally present with peracute or acute onset of neurologic deficits. Decompressive surgery is indicated in some of these patients. Physiotherapy typically focuses on intensive pain management and supportive care immediately after surgery, transitioning fairly quickly to an emphasis on promoting mobility and supporting a return to function. Although recovery times may vary greatly, the first 2 to 4 weeks of the recovery period are the most illuminating with regard to the patient's long-term prognosis.[10] For most patients, major milestones of recovery such as the restoration of deep pain sensation and return of voluntary motor function occur during that early time period. Still, recovery is slower in more severely affected patients. Time to return of motor function can be as long as 9 months after surgery or injury.[10] For patients that do not regain the ability to walk in the first month or two, supportive care and physiotherapy to manage the secondary effects of their disease is of even greater importance; however, the costs of care may dictate that a greater proportion of the therapy program be conducted by the client at home. For these patients, a mobility aid such as an ambulation cart may significantly improve quality of life and decrease the risk of secondary complications from immobility.

Spinal cord diseases such as Hansen type II intervertebral disc disease and degenerative myelopathy are typically associated with more chronic, slowly progressive neurologic deficits. These more chronic conditions warrant a different therapeutic approach with less emphasis on aggressive management in the near term and a greater focus on frequent repetition of low-impact and low-intensity activities to preserve neuromuscular and musculoskeletal function, and long-term pain management in some patients. Regular physiotherapy for patients with presumptive degenerative myelopathy has been associated with longer survival times.[11]

PHYSIOTHERAPY FOR DISEASES OF THE PERIPHERAL NEUROMUSCULAR SYSTEM

There are a wide variety of diseases that can affect the peripheral nervous system (PNS). The main components of the PNS are muscle, the neuromuscular junction, and peripheral nerve. Neurologic examination findings in patients with PNS disease are variable, depending on which component is affected and the underlying etiology; therefore, a thorough diagnostic workup is necessary. Broad etiologic categories of PNS disease include degenerative, metabolic, inflammatory, neoplastic, and toxic. Although the mainstay of management for many neuromuscular diseases is treatment of the primary underlying condition (ie, diabetic neuropathy, paraneoplastic neuropathy), physiotherapy should be considered an important adjunctive therapy. Patients with lower motor neuron tetraparesis/tetraplegia caused by diseases such as botulism and acute canine polyradiculoneuritis often experience a prolonged recovery lasting weeks to months, during which physical therapy and appropriate supportive care is essential. Physiotherapy may also be incorporated into the treatment plan of those patients affected by chronic, progressive, degenerative polyneuropathies to preserve muscle mass and maintain strength. However, further investigation is necessary to determine whether physical therapy truly slows the progression of disease. In humans, strength and balance training is safe and effective for patients with peripheral neuropathy.[12]

PHYSIOTHERAPY OF INTRACRANIAL DISEASE

Although intracranial diseases are managed extensively with physical therapy in human medicine,[13–15] this field remains essentially unexplored in veterinary rehabilitation. Anecdotal successes have been achieved in various clinical scenarios; however, clinical trials evaluating the use of physiotherapy for the management of intracranial disease in dogs and cats have not been reported, to our knowledge.

CARE OF NEUROLOGIC PATIENTS
Supportive Care

Supportive care and nursing care are central to the physiotherapy plan of neurologic patients. Many patients with neurologic illness are severely debilitated on initial presentation. Patients should be clinically stable before starting a physiotherapy program, with all critical surgical and medical needs addressed. Although sometimes overlooked, a key treatment objective is supportive care to prevent or mitigate secondary complications. Appropriate nursing care, particularly of the urinary, dermatologic, and pulmonary systems, is imperative for the prevention and management of decubitus ulcers, urine scalding, and infection. The likelihood of developing 1 or more of these complications is increased by the presence of comorbidities such as obesity, an endocrinopathy, or physical trauma to other body systems, which must be identified and appropriately managed. The role of the technical staff in management of a recumbent patient is absolutely critical. It is therefore important that all staff tasked with the care of neurologic patients have appropriate training and are aware of the potential deleterious effects of inadequate care.

Bedding and harnesses

Immobile and nonambulatory patients must be provided with adequate bedding. Ideally, bedding should be smooth, stable, nonporous (or easily cleaned and replaced), and deformable, yet also act to disburse the patient's weight over a large surface area. Patients should be monitored closely and checked frequently (sometimes as often as hourly) for soiling. Bedding that is wet with water, urine, feces, or serous and purulent discharge needs to be replaced immediately. Because the patient's skin may require frequent cleaning, detergents and materials used for cleaning should be gentle products that will not disrupt the protective epidermal layer. Patients that are not yet able to hold themselves in a sternal position, or who lay preferentially on 1 side or the other should be turned every 4 to 6 hours with adequate notations made in the treatment notes. Bedding specifically intended to avoid decubitus ulcers is commercially available (Kloud9, Vivorté, Louisville, KY, USA).

Managing the large recumbent patient presents unique practical challenges. Larger patients, whether they are obese or large breed dogs of appropriate body condition, are at increased risk of pressure necrosis of the skin (also known as decubitus ulcers or bed sores), compartment syndrome, and lung atelectasis simply owing to their greater weight. Obese patients may be predisposed to infection owing to chronic metabolic stress resulting from obesity and increased resistance to peripheral circulation in proportion to the amount of adipose tissue present. These patients require particularly close monitoring, and should be turned from side to side more frequently to prevent these complications. Turning large, severely debilitated patients without risk of injury to the patient or staff may require the use of assistive devices like a hoist or a sling.

A variety of devices are available to assist in the support and mobilization of large patients. A hoist (Hoyer lift) can be adapted for veterinary patients with an appropriately designed harness (**Fig. 1**). Hoyer lifts are manual (hydraulic) or battery powered. Hydraulic lifts do not require charging before use and are more tolerant of extended storage periods. Electric or battery-powered models require less effort to operate than manual models; however, they are more expensive to purchase and maintain. Care should be taken that the harness used with a Hoyer lift distributes the patient's weight evenly and does not place undue stress over a particular region, particularly the urinary bladder. Most Hoyer lifts have wheels, although they can be awkward to maneuver over long distances. Several companies commercialize adjustable wheeled "quad" carts that can be used in the hospital setting to facilitate patient mobility and allow the patient to eat or walk in a standing position (**Fig. 2**). A quad cart is

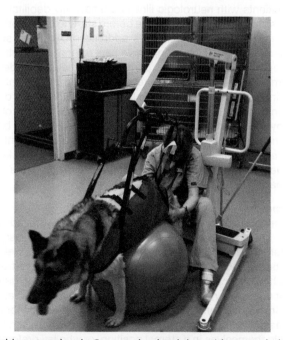

Fig. 1. A 7-year-old neutered male German shepherd dog with nonambulatory paraparesis after intervertebral disc herniation and hemilaminectomy is standing with his weight supported by a hoist and an exercise ball. The therapist places his pelvic limb in a weight-bearing position and performs a gentle weight-shifting exercise.

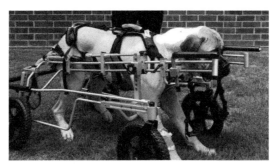

Fig. 2. A 3.5-year-old castrated male Mastiff with nonambulatory tetraparesis 7 days after multilevel dorsal laminectomy to correct cervical spondylomyelopathy is standing in an Eddie's Wheels Adjustable clinic quad cart (Eddie's Wheels, Shelburne Falls, MA; with permission.) The cart's width, length, and height have been adjusted to fit the patient.

generally more maneuverable than a Hoyer lift; however, many have a maximum weight limit of 70 to 90 kg (150–200 lbs) and are not suitable for the largest dogs, or for species other than dogs.

Harnesses are available to assist in lifting heavy patients and to support mobility until the patient regains sufficient strength and coordination to be independently ambulatory (Help'Em Up, Blue Dog Designs, Denver, CO, USA). Because the majority of neurologically impaired patients in the rehabilitation setting are affected primarily or only in the rear legs, harnesses that provide pelvic support are essential for neurologic rehabilitation. The harness should be constructed of durable yet soft, lightweight, and breathable material with smooth or padded edges to prevent rubbing or pinching of the skin and catching of the fur. When the patient's weight is fully supported, there should not be any focal areas of pressure or restriction that limit circulation or cause tissue injury. Seams and attachments such as handles or metal rings should be secure and sturdy enough to withstand significant and repeated strains. Harnesses will become soiled and need to be tolerant of frequent hand or machine washing with sanitizing detergents. It is helpful to have a supply of harnesses available for clients to rent or purchase for use at home as well. Clients should be advised on how to clean and maintain the harness and to monitor the pet closely for signs of abrasion or infection at points of contact with the skin.

Pressure sores, abrasions, and decubitus ulcers

Skin lesions are common complications of recumbency. They range from erythema to full-thickness skin necrosis (**Fig. 3**). Areas of pressure necrosis or decubital ulceration must be managed aggressively to prevent infection and enlargement of the primary lesion. Decubital ulcers can develop rapidly, especially when early signs of devitalization are overlooked. As a precaution, any areas of hair loss, erythema, contusion, or abrasion should be assumed to be incipient pressure necrosis. Additional padding should be applied around these areas to limit direct contact with bedding or pressure points, and lesions should be monitored daily for evidence of progression. Similarly, patients should be monitored regularly for signs of emergent infection. Treatment for any developing infection is implemented as soon as is practical. Although not always possible, antibiotic therapy should be guided by culture and susceptibility of an appropriate tissue or fluid sample. For tissue necrosis with or without tissue sloughing, bandaging these areas with several layers of pliable, absorbent material may help to prevent further trauma. Bandages should be replaced at least once daily, and more

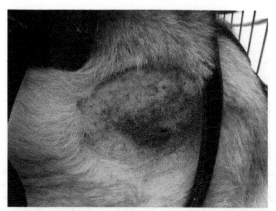

Fig. 3. A 13-year-old German Shepherd dog was nonambulatory paraparetic with multifocal type II intervertebral disc disease. The dog developed skin lesions associated with his prolonged recumbency. A full-thickness ulcer is present over the greater trochanter. The skin is edematous and erythematous proximal to the ulcer.

often when there is significant exudate from the wound or soiling from external sources. In areas where bandaging is not feasible or practical, providing additional padding around the wound margins with a central area of noncontact (as with a "doughnut" ring) can relieve the pressure on the wound and also allow increased air flow. When the lesions are asymmetrical, patients should be encouraged to spend more time resting on the unaffected side. Exposed wounds can be soaked or washed gently with an antiseptic solution (ie, 0.05% chlorhexidine diacetate; Nolvasan, Zoetis, Florham Park, NJ, USA) every few hours to prevent contamination and aid with debridement; however, these areas should be allowed to dry completely between treatments. Because ensuring timely resolution of wounds is particularly important in the hospital setting, it is worthwhile to consider the use of additional modalities to speed the healing process and prevent indolence. The use of therapeutic ultrasonography to speed wound healing is well established.[16] Similarly, low-level laser therapy may be useful, although this technology seems to be less substantiated.

Patients with diminished or absent proprioception and sensory capacity are prone to the development of skin lesions ranging from hair loss and abrasions to full-thickness wounds on the digits and bony prominences of the lower limbs owing to pressure necrosis, to scuffing on the ground, or to self-mutilation (**Fig. 4**). As with pressure necrosis lesions, abrasions on the extremities can quickly progress to full-thickness lesions and may develop infection from bacterial contamination. The toes and distal limbs can be protected from trauma with the use of bandages or commercial booties (Walkaboots, Thera-Paw, Lebanon, NJ, USA; or Summit Trex, Ruffwear, Bend, OR, USA). The bootie should also fit securely but not constrict the thin, soft tissue layers of the extremities. The use of booties can be problematic because those that provide adequate protection to the skin may limit sensory input to the distal limb, potentially hindering any emerging proprioceptive signaling. Also, the weight of the bootie may complicate locomotion in dogs with weak hock flexion secondary to sciatic neuropathy or weak carpal extension secondary to radial nerve palsy. Many patients will object to the feel of the booties or be inclined to chew at the unfamiliar article. Bootie selection should be made with an understanding of these considerations.

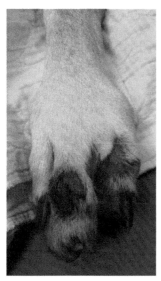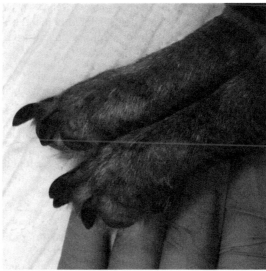

Fig. 4. Dogs with sciatic neuropathy are vulnerable to skin abrasions over phalanges (*left*) and the metatarsal region (*right*). The dog on the left has a full-thickness wound on the third digit and a superficial abrasion of the fifth digit. The dog on the right has partial thickness wounds on the lateral aspect of the fifth metatarsal bone.

For patients with some motor function that still require assistance with traction and proprioception, alternatives to a heavy protective bootie may be more appropriate. Devices that lift the hock or digits or both to prevent wear (**Fig. 5**) can be quite useful for short periods to help facilitate therapeutic exercises or make leash walking at home feasible (Anti-Knuckling Device, Canine Mobility, Seattle, WA, USA; or Biko Mobility, Raleigh, NC, USA). Similarly, thin rubber coverings for the paw or rubber grips placed on the toenails may allow greater sensory input while still providing traction (Toe Grips,

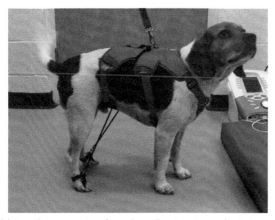

Fig. 5. A 4-year-old Beagle recovering from hemilaminectomy for intervertebral disc herniation at T13–L1 and L1–L2 is wearing elastic bands to correct a residual proprioceptive deficit. The elastic bands connect the phalanges and metatarsus to a chest harness. Tension in the bands promotes extension of the digits and eliminates scuffing at a walk and trot.

Dr Buzby's ToeGrips for Dogs, Beaufort, SC, USA). Nonporous coverings (Pawz; available: http://pawzdogboots.com/) should be used only during supervised activity and for short periods of time to prevent the patient from ingesting the material or developing pododermatitis.

Bladder management

Many patients with spinal cord disease also have bladder and urethral dysfunction. In the rehabilitation setting, patients should be monitored continuously for signs of urinary tract injury or compromise. When the patient is completely unable to initiate or complete micturition, the bladder needs to be manually expressed (**Fig. 6**) or catheterized every 6 to 8 hours to ensure complete emptying. Patients on fluid therapy require more frequent emptying. As the patient regains function, and particularly once there is indication of returning voluntary motor function, the frequency of manual expression may be decreased. In many instances, bladder management may be facilitated with the use of medications such as oral diazepam (0.25–0.5 mg/kg every 8–12 hours), phenoxybenzamine (0.25–0.5 mg/kg every 8–12 hours), and rarely, bethanechol (2.5–15 mg, total dose, PO q8 hours).[17] Urinary tract infection is a leading complication of recumbency.[18] Owners of patients managed as outpatients should be advised to watch for any change in the frequency or amount of urine production, changes in color or odor, and the presence of blood, fibrin, or mucus. Even when no outward signs of infection are present, and especially for patients using the underwater treadmill, routine monitoring is recommended, with serial urine cultures every 4 to 6 weeks initially and then every 3 months once the patient's neurologic status has stabilized, for as long as they remain nonambulatory. For hospitalized patients, empiric antibiotic therapy without culture and sensitivity is not recommended to avoid promoting antimicrobial resistance.

Other supportive care considerations

Patients with neurologic impairment frequently also experience fecal incontinence, for which medical management options are limited. For these patients, appropriate sanitation and nursing care as described are the primary management goals. The perianal and perineal skin of patients with fecal incontinence should be monitored carefully for evidence of scalding, ulceration, or infection. Application of a moisture barrier cream (eg, zinc-based diaper cream, commercial antiseptics such as Calmoseptine [Huntington Beach, CA, USA]) may be helpful in preserving skin integrity and preventing contamination.

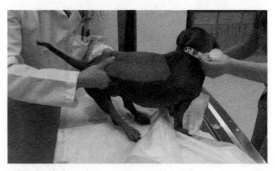

Fig. 6. A 4.5-year-old Dachshund is paraparetic with upper motor neuron bladder dysfunction after a T12–T13 disc herniation and hemilaminectomy. The urine is expressed by placing pressure on the bladder using 2 hands.

THE PHYSIOTHERAPY PLAN

A comprehensive physiotherapy plan aims to manage pain, prevent secondary complications of immobility, and support the health and function of the musculoskeletal tissues during the recovery process. Neurologically impaired patients range in ability from complete immobility or tetraplegia/paraplegia, through tetraparesis/paraparesis, to mild ataxia, or even pain only. Patients may present for therapy at any point during the clinical course of disease and the same patient may pass through several stages over the course of his or her recovery. For postsurgical patients or patients with persistent spinal instability, the physiotherapist and therapy assistants should protect the site of injury when designing and enacting the treatment plan. Other important considerations for the design of a physiotherapy program include access to the patient, level of staff support, and the safety of staff, patient and client when performing treatments. **Table 1** lists a number of factors that influence the rehabilitation plan. For cases with a significant number of limitations or complicating factors, it may be wise to consider inpatient care or referral to a specialty facility with a rehabilitation therapist on staff.

Because patient cooperation is key to any rehabilitation therapy plan, particularly one that is to be carried out primarily at home by the owner, efforts should be made to ensure that the prescribed treatments cause minimal stress or discomfort for the patient. This is a significant departure from the philosophy of some aspects of physical therapy in humans. A physiotherapy program that is painful or stressful for the patient is unlikely to be effective, may cause the patient to become aggressive, and will potentially damage the human–animal bond between client and patient. To minimize stress, treatments should, whenever possible, be administered in a calm environment using equipment or activities that are already familiar to the patient. New equipment or activities should be introduced gradually with a period of acclimatization. Therapies should limit or avoid causing pain or fatigue.

Passive Manual Therapy

Passive range of motion (PROM) activities are commonly prescribed for neurologically impaired patients. PROM involves the use of external forces applied to the limbs or

Table 1			
Factors affecting the rehabilitation therapy program design			
Patient Factors	**Client Factors**	**Facility Factors**	**Staff Factors**
Size	Physical abilities	Size and indoor or outdoor exercise space	Availability of sufficient support staff
Temperament	Financial resources	Availability of lift equipment	Proper training and experience
Degree of disability	Schedule and household restrictions	Appropriate modalities	Physical ability to lift and transport patients
Location of incision(s)	Emotional needs and concerns	Facility hours	Access to specialists
Intravenous or urinary catheterization		Adequate bedding and housing	
Bandages and external coaptation			
Comorbidities			

axial skeleton to flex and extend joints when the patient is -plegic or too weak to effect active range of motion. PROM is frequently combined with stretching of the periarticular connective tissues and skeletal muscle. The primary benefit of PROM is protection against stiffening or fibrosis of the joint. Other benefits may include prevention of cartilage atrophy, replenishment of the synovial fluid (primary source of nutrients for the cartilage), improved local circulation, and stimulation of sensory and proprioceptive pathways in the synovium and periarticular structures. Although frequently prescribed and simple in concept, PROM can be misapplied or performed incorrectly. It is important that an appropriate technique be used to achieve maximum benefit and prevent injury to the animal, whether this treatment is administered by the hospital staff or by the client at home. PROM should be performed with a patient that is relaxed and cooperative. The limb should be gripped firmly but gently and the motion performed along the normal plane of limb movement during ambulation with the long bones in proper alignment to each other. Each cycle should be performed smoothly and deliberately. It is not necessary to reach maximum flexion or extension for the activity to be effective. Rather, the movement should only be performed in the range that the patient is comfortable and does not resist. Owners in particular may have a tendency to want to force the leg in 1 direction or the other, which may cause tissue strain and will also result in a stressful experience for the patient and a loss of trust that will make other treatment sessions more difficult.

Massage is another passive therapy with multiple benefits. In humans, there is evidence that massage therapy alleviates pain and stress associated with recent injury or surgery.[19] Massage also improves both local and whole-body circulation and lymphatic drainage, allowing for increased tissue oxygenation and more rapid resolution of edema.[20] For patients experiencing muscle tremors, spasms, or rigidity, massage can provide transient relief of these symptoms. In addition, massage provides additional sensory stimulation that may encourage nerve regeneration in the affected tissues. Massage is clearly pleasurable for the majority of rehabilitation patients and beginning a therapy session with a whole-body massage in a calming environment may improve patient compliance thereby increasing the effectiveness of the therapy program. Massage techniques vary depending on the preference and training of the therapist and may need to be adjusted based on a patient's level of sensitivity or tolerance. A number of lay publications describe massage techniques in some detail. These may be useful resources for clients when massage is prescribed as a part of the home therapy plan. In general, massage for patients with neurologic disease requires only light pressure applied in long strokes or circular motions. Massage may be applied only to the affected limbs or to the entire body. For patients that are primarily affected in their hind limbs and carrying an atypical proportion of their weight on the forelegs, massage may relieve secondary muscle strain in the neck and shoulders. Gentle massage adjacent to the site of surgery or injury may help to relieve muscle tension and inflammation in this area as well, although direct pressure over the surgical incision or an area that is persistently unstable is inadvisable.

Acupuncture is categorized here as a passive manual therapy because it does not require the active involvement of the patient and relies primarily on direct mechanical stimulation to achieve its effects. The scientific literature is mixed regarding the therapeutic benefits of acupuncture overall, but the evidence may be more encouraging when examining the benefits of acupuncture specifically for neurogenic pain and the facilitation of nerve signaling.[21,22] Acupuncture has been demonstrated to increase serotonin levels in the serum and cerebrospinal fluid of both human and canine patients. Because it is a noninvasive technique with limited potential for adverse effects, acupuncture is often utilized as a component of the neurologic physiotherapy program, but rarely as a sole therapy. Unfortunately, this very ubiquity as an adjunctive treatment and a lack of controlled studies evaluating acupuncture as a sole therapy make it difficult to determine what definite value, if any, acupuncture provides.

Therapeutic Exercises

Although there are several therapeutic exercises useful for patients with varying degrees of mobility and strength, the level of difficulty and amount of assistance provided for any given activity is always adjusted according to the clinical status of each patient. When selecting specific exercises for the therapy program, some thought must be given to the muscle groups and anatomic regions that will be involved in performing the exercise and in particular any areas that may experience strain or weakness during the activity. Exercise therapy plays a crucial role in any physiotherapy program, and especially so with neurologic patients. Targeted exercise therapy aids in the management or prevention of many of the consequences of immobility, including atrophy of soft and bony tissues, stiffening or fibrosis, maintaining proper proteoglycan matrix in the articular cartilage, and stimulating the synovium to replenish the joint fluid. Exercise therapy stimulates transmission of nerve signals, reinforces proprioceptive and motor pathways, and aids in the restoration of muscle memory for standing, walking, and other activities that require minimal or no conscious effort in the healthy patient. There are many specific exercises that can be used in the course of a rehabilitation program. As long as the prescribed exercises are safe and appropriate for the given patient's physical and medical status, the therapist is limited only by his or her own creativity. Clients are often an excellent resource for conceiving exercises that dovetail with the patient's current routine and level of training and it is generally helpful to include them in the process of developing the exercise program. In many instances, as patients recover from neurologic injury, they experience the greatest difficulty with transitions from 1 position or activity to another (eg, lateral to sternal recumbency, sitting to standing, making turns, and stepping over obstacles). Exercises that aid in development or preservation of the core muscle groups along the spine and abdomen are particularly helpful in improving a patient's ability to handle these transitional movements.

Exercise therapy for the nonambulatory patient

Recumbent patients should be assisted into a sternal position with the limbs placed appropriately to either side for brief periods intermittently throughout the day. The patient should be encouraged to remain in this position for as long as possible at each attempt. Support can be offered using the therapist's hands, wedge cushions, a harness, or other device (eg, gallon jugs filled with sand placed along the chest) and should be provided only to the degree necessary for the animal to remain in the desired position. As strength returns, the amount of support is incrementally reduced until the patient is able to maintain sternal recumbency unassisted. At this stage, placing the patent on a less supportive surface such as a well-stabilized wobble board or therapy ball can increase the degree of difficulty.

As soon as the patient achieves sufficient tone to allow for assisted standing, therapy sessions should incorporate brief periods with the patient in a standing position, with gradually diminishing support and increasing difficulty, as noted. Gentle weight-shifting activities may also be introduced at this stage. To promote normal motor signaling and muscle memory, the patient should be positioned in a way that approximates a normal standing posture as closely as possible, including the spacing of the paws under the body and distribution of weight to all legs. For any supported postural activity, care should be taken to maintain normal spinal alignment and avoid torsion, distraction, compression, or bending of the spine, particularly at the site of injury or surgery. Once the patient is able to stand unassisted for several seconds, the therapist may begin assisted sitting exercises, taking care to always begin with the patient in a correct sitting posture. As described, this activity can be made increasingly difficult using a wobble board or balance disk. The exercise program is gradually adjusted to increase the degree of difficulty according to the patient's level of function.

Aquatic therapy, when available, is an important component of the therapeutic exercise program. Standing in water is a very comfortable form of assisted stance for nonambulatory patients (**Fig. 7**). Underwater exercise, whether walking on a treadmill or swimming, yields limb movements earlier in the recovery period than exercise on dry land. There are numerous benefits to the performance of exercise while partially or completely submerged in water. Among these is the quality of buoyancy, which minimizes the weight-bearing load on the joints, decreasing the pain associated with movement.[23] The resistance of the water maximizes the effect of exertion on the muscles, allowing for greater strengthening with minimal activity. Resistance also slows movement, allowing for greater reaction time, and providing an opportunity for proper foot placement, thereby reinforcing a proper gait pattern and proprioceptive signaling. Buoyancy and resistance promote increased range of motion in specific joints during underwater activities. Walking on an underwater treadmill is a more controlled movement than swimming, placing less strain or torque on the spine and joints and thus may be more appropriate for the early stages of recovery and strength building. Other properties of water are also beneficial for patients experiencing prolonged immobility or weakness, including hydrostatic pressure that helps to reduce edema and promote lymphatic drainage. The temperature of the water is kept comfortably warm, further promoting blood circulation and lymphatic drainage. In humans, underwater exercise has been shown to be less taxing on the cardiovascular and respiratory systems, which is helpful for obese patients or those with concurrent illness.[24]

Exercise therapy for the ambulatory patient

As patients regain function or for ambulatory patients, exercises to reinforce muscle strength, balance, and proprioception take on an important role in the rehabilitation program. Ambulation assistance by means of a harness can be conveniently provided when a dog walks on a treadmill (**Fig. 8**). Once the dog can walk independently, land-based activities such as walking over textured or yielding surfaces, Cavaletti rails, weaving, inclines, leg weights, and low steps are introduced singly or in combination

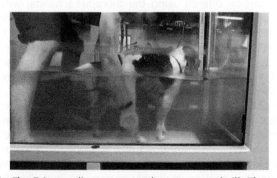

Fig. 7. The dog in **Fig. 5** is standing on an underwater treadmill. The water supports his weight. The therapist is placing his pelvic limbs in a weight-bearing position and doing a gentle weight shifting exercise.

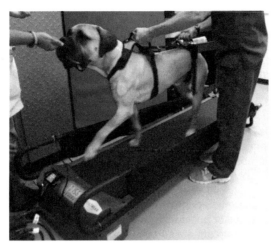

Fig. 8. The dog seen in **Fig. 2** is seen 28 days after multilevel dorsal laminectomy for cervical spondylomyelopathy. The dog is walking on a treadmill at an incline while being supported and controlled by a harness.

to promote strength, flexibility, and coordination. The design of each activity should be calibrated to the ability and inclination of the patient.

Electrophysical Modalities

Several of the modalities available to the rehabilitation practitioner may be useful in enhancing the physiotherapy plan. Although an extensive review of the technology, mechanism of action, and application of the available modalities is beyond the scope of this article, a brief review is presented herein. Please refer to the references for more details.

Low-level laser therapy

Low-level laser therapy has been demonstrated to accelerate wound healing in human patients, particularly those with metabolic or physical compromise that may delay normal wound healing.[25,26] In the hospital environment, where rapid and complete resolution of any skin wounds is desirable to reduce the risk of nosocomial infection, the application of laser light therapy to areas of inflamed, devitalized, or abraded skin is a reasonable adjunct to standard wound management. Furthermore, laser may have direct beneficial effects on nerve cells and their supporting structures. Preliminary work suggests that daily therapy with 810 nm light over the surgical site in the 5 to 7 days after hemilaminectomy reduces the time to ambulation by 7 days on average. Although the mechanism of action for therapeutic laser has yet to be fully characterized, it is generally accepted that laser can act to increase the production of cellular adenosine triphosphate at the mitochondrial level by stimulating light-receptive molecules (chromophores) in the mitochondrial membrane. Treatment dose is most commonly measured as a unit of energy (eg, Joules per square centimeter of skin exposed to the laser light). The total dose can be adjusted by increasing or decreasing treatment time or intensity (Watts.) Most commercially available therapeutic lasers emit 3 or 4 separate wavelengths ranging from 600 to 1000 nm. The specific wavelengths of devices vary by manufacturer and there is no evidence documenting the most effective wavelength or dose for tissue types or disease conditions. Tissue penetration is largely determined by wavelength (deeper penetration is achieved by longer wavelengths), although this is influenced by treatment intensity and skin color. Dose ranges for standard treatments typically range from 1 to 4 J/cm^2 for superficial tissues with lower protein levels (dermis, epidermis) and from 8 to 12 J/cm^2 for deeper tissues or tissues with higher protein content. There is increasing evidence in the literature that cells may be most responsive to moderate doses of phototherapy. Higher doses seem to not only fail to improve the therapeutic outcome, but in some cases may actually inhibit the desired tissue response. As recovery progresses, frequency of laser treatment is reduced accordingly. Currently, there is debate surrounding the question of tissue penetration with phototherapy. As much as 66% of percutaneous laser light energy is absorbed or scattered in the first 2 mm of human skin.[27] The remaining dose probably does not penetrate more than 1 to 2 cm as monochromatic, collimated and coherent light energy. Tissue type and species of the patient may significantly affect penetration depths. Depth of penetration may improve with more prolonged exposure times or pulsed therapy, suggesting a possible advantage to using lower intensity, pulsed treatment settings applied over a longer treatment time. For medium- and large-breed dogs with spinal cord injury, it is unlikely that percutaneous laser light is actually delivered to the injured tissue in its original form. It is unknown whether the light must retain the properties of collimation and coherence to stimulate an effect at the level of the chromophore. In the case of spinal cord injury, the benefits of laser therapy may derive from regional and systemic effects rather than via direct influence on the injured nervous system tissue. When applied at higher intensities or for too long over a given area, low-level laser can cause thermal damage and phototoxicity to the tissues.

Therapeutic ultrasonography

Therapeutic ultrasonography is beneficial for patients with joint stiffening, connective tissue trauma, or muscle spasm. The therapeutic effects of ultrasound therapy may derive primarily from tissue heating and increased collagen elasticity. Continuous ultrasound therapy has a heating effect on soft tissues at greater depths (2–5 cm) than external heat sources (1–2 cm). As with other forms of thermotherapy, a change in tissue temperature of 2°C to 4°C increases local blood flow and tissue extensibility while also reducing muscle spasm. These effects provide pain relief and are useful in conjunction with a stretching program to preserve or restore joint flexibility or prevent skeletal muscle contracture and fibrosis. Sound waves are delivered through probes of varying diameters ranging from 1 to 10 cm^2 depending on the size and contour of the area being treated. Heads measuring 5 cm^2 are used most commonly. Ultrasound intensity is measured in watts per square centimeter. Treatment intensities vary with the type of tissue being treated (tissues with higher protein content absorb more sound energy) and the treatment indication. Most therapeutic ultrasound machines have adjustable wavelengths. Longer wavelengths are used for superficial applications. Treatment time is 3 to 4 minutes for each ultrasound head for a total treatment time of 4 to 10 minutes. Treatment times of approximately 4 minutes seem sufficient to generate the desired tissue temperature increase. Areas greater than 10 cm^2 should be divided into sections with each section treated independently because dissipation of the sound energy over too large an area may result in inadequate thermal change. Therapeutic ultrasonography can be administered once or twice daily for patients with intense pain or spasm. Patients that are not as severely affected require fewer treatments. Therapeutic ultrasonography may also be beneficial at nonthermal (interrupted duty cycle) settings. The benefits of this modality in promoting tissue healing are well established and have been applied to management of skin wounds, skeletal muscle tears, tendon and ligament rupture, and bone healing (as with nonunion fractures).[28] The sound waves generated by therapeutic ultrasonography, like those used for diagnostic ultrasonography, do not transmit effectively through air, although air and other gas interfaces will experience some of the same thermal effects as soft tissue. To maximize the transmission of ultrasonography to the target tissue and improve patient comfort, ultrasound therapy should be applied over skin that is clipped or shaved and clean. The use of a transducer gel is necessary to maximize contact and eliminate gas interference between the ultrasound head and the skin surface.

Electrical stimulation

Electrical stimulation has 2 major applications for the patient with neurologic disease or impairment. Neuromuscular electrical nerve stimulation (NMES) involves the administration of an electrical impulse across skeletal muscle tissue to stimulate a contraction when voluntary motor function is absent or weak. In NMES, electrode pads are placed on the skin and the electrical impulse is delivered percutaneously (**Fig. 9**). Electrical muscle stimulation is a variation on NMES where needle-shaped electrodes are inserted directly into the muscle. Because electrical muscle stimulation is a more invasive technique and requires greater precision in electrode placement, it is not commonly performed in the clinical rehabilitation therapy setting. Although NMES does not recruit muscle fibers in the same sequence, nor to the same degree as voluntary movement, it can be used to preserve the integrity and mass of muscle fibers and prevent atrophy secondary to disuse. It can also be used in the case of denervation injury; however, it must be administered daily and may be of little value in the case of complete denervation when motor function is unlikely to be restored, because it slows muscle atrophy but does not change the outcome of denervation. To generate effective muscle contractions, 1 electrode is placed near the motor point of the muscle and the other is placed along the muscle body. Motor points are typically near the origin of the muscle. Once the placement of the electrodes has been confirmed and a perceptible muscle contraction elicited, the electrical stimulation should be cycled so that periods of contraction are separated by periods of rest at approximately a

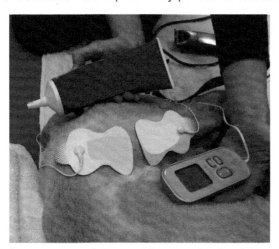

Fig. 9. A nonambulatory, paraparetic 7-year-old castrated male mix-breed dog is receiving neuromuscular electrical stimulation of his left quadriceps femoris muscle to increase muscle mass. The thigh was clipped. The proximal electrode is applied near the motor point of the quadriceps. The distal electrode is applied on the distal portion of the muscle.

1:2 to 1:5 ratio, based on muscle fitness. Treatment settings for NMES, particularly intensity, may vary from patient to patient and even between treatment sessions on the same patient. A variety of waveforms can be used for NMES therapy, although a symmetric biphasic form seems to be best tolerated (eg, variable muscle stimulation [VMS]). Generally, pulse frequency should be adjusted upward until the contractions are smooth and well tolerated. Lower pulse frequencies result in a more perceptible contraction because the muscle visibly "pulses" with a regular beat. However, this pulsing beat may be uncomfortable, even when sensory perception is otherwise diminished. The intensity of the electrical stimulation (most often measured in volts or milliamperes) is adjusted upward until the strongest contraction is elicited or to the highest level that the patient will tolerate and then decreased slightly to achieve the appropriate setting. The treatment period should last 10 to 20 minutes, or until there is perceptible fatigue of the muscle. Treatments should be administered daily (or as often as possible if daily therapy is not feasible) until voluntary motor function is restored.

In transcutaneous electrical nerve stimulation (TENS), electrodes are placed at points that bracket the area of inflammation or pain, and electrical impulses travel through that area. TENS therapy has a primary goal of pain relief rather than muscle contraction. TENS therapy may also reduce edema, increase perfusion, speed tissue healing, and attract certain inflammatory cell types to the affected area.[29,30] As with NMES, treatment settings are not established by formula and are frequently based primarily on the therapist's assessment of patient comfort and tolerance. Higher frequencies are often better tolerated. Intensity is generally increased gradually over the first 3 to 5 minutes until a response is elicited from the patient. If the patient is comfortable, the intensity is maintained at that level for the duration of the treatment. If the patient shows signs of discomfort, the intensity may be decreased slightly until it is well tolerated. A treatment period of 40 minutes provides optimal pain management.[31] Pain relief after TENS may last up to 4 days. When used as an adjunct or sole therapy for pain management, TENS treatments should be administered as frequently as necessary to keep the patient comfortable, typically once every 24 to 48 hours, initially. Many clients are familiar with TENS therapy from personal experience and some have TENS units of their own at home. Although it is not unreasonable to prescribe TENS therapy for clients to administer at home, clients may encounter variable success, even with careful coaching. Because electrical stimulation can cause significant patient discomfort when misapplied, leading to an aversion to therapeutic interventions and decreased patient compliance, it may be wise to restrict the use of TENS to the clinical setting, with exceptions. With any electrical stimulation technique, electrodes should be applied to skin that has been clipped and cleaned. Preparation of the skin by swabbing with rubbing alcohol to remove surface oils is helpful. Although the risk of combustion is low, rubbing alcohol or other solvents should be allowed to dry thoroughly before initiation of the electrical stimulation to reduce the risk of tissue burns. A transducer gel can be applied to the skin under the electrode pad to improve conduction of the electrical impulse and patient comfort. Although the transducer gels used for standard ultrasound therapy may be effective for electrical stimulation, a gel specifically designed to promote electrical conduction, such as the Spectra 360 brand (Parker Laboratories, Fairfield, NJ, USA) is recommended.

CLIENT EDUCATION AND SUPPORT DURING HOME THERAPY

The importance of client education and support for owners of neurologically impaired patients was mentioned earlier in this article. The physiotherapist plays a key role in teaching the client how to manage the needs of a patient with limited mobility, possibly more so than any other clinician involved in the medical management of patients with neurologic injury or disease. Regardless of how thorough the professional physio-therapy and medical management program, owners bear the greatest responsibility for patient care once discharged from the hospital. Clients should be informed about the patient's nursing care needs and signs of complications that need to be addressed by their primary veterinarian. A thorough description, ideally with visual or written aids, of any home physiotherapy treatments will improve the client's confidence and in-crease compliance.

When prescribing a home care plan, the therapist must evaluate the owner's ability to understand and safely perform the recommended treatments. Similarly, financial, physical, or scheduling restrictions facing the client or pet in the home environment should be discussed because they impact the type, number, and frequency of any prescribed treatments. In cases where the family schedule or home environment cannot accommodate the needs of the patient in the near term, the therapist may recommend hospitalizing or boarding the patient for inpatient care during the initial phases of the physiotherapy program. The use of readily available or inexpensive ma-terials minimizes the burden on the client to seek out or develop equipment for their pet's therapy.

A thorough overview of the treatment plan and expected outcome should be dis-cussed with the client at the onset of therapy and reviewed frequently, particularly as the patient's status changes. It is important to include information such as a description or demonstration of the activities to be performed, how frequently the treatments should be performed, signs that indicate a treatment is not well tolerated or ineffective, a basic understanding of relevant anatomy and an approximate time-line for the anticipated results. It is often helpful to give clients both short-term and long-term goals so that they understand the anticipated progression of the patient and they have realistic expectations. The physiotherapist is often the client's most frequent point of contact over the course of treatment and should be prepared not only to provide guidance on medical and nursing care, but also to address concerns related to patient welfare, related to the emotional, physical, and financial burdens of managing a pet with special needs, and related to quality-of-life and end-of-life decisions. Many clients are overwhelmed with the degree of their pet's disability and the tremendous impact of their care on the home routine. Often, cli-ents do not reach a full realization of their new responsibilities until several days or weeks after the diagnosis is obtained and the patient is discharged from the hos-pital. The rehabilitation therapist can help the client to set realistic expectations for the timing and extent of recovery or, in the case of degenerative diseases, the rate of decline. The therapist should strive to be neither overly optimistic nor overly doubtful with regard to the patient's prognosis. It is useful to build a relationship with a counselor or therapist with experience in managing the needs of families experiencing major illness or life-changing disability. Clients will greatly benefit from referral to a therapist who can help manage the emotional fallout from caring for a paralyzed or debilitated pet.

REFERENCES

1. Forterre F, Gorgas D, Dickomeit M, et al. Incidence of spinal compressive lesions in chondrodystrophic dogs with abnormal recovery after hemilaminectomy for treatment of thoracolumbar disc disease: a prospective magnetic resonance im-aging study. Vet Surg 2010;39:165–72.

2. Parent J. Clinical approach and lesion localization in patients with spinal diseases. Vet Clin North Am Small Anim Pract 2010;40:733–53.
3. Olby NJ, De Risio L, Munana KR, et al. Development of a functional scoring system in dogs with acute spinal cord injuries. Am J Vet Res 2001;62:1624–8.
4. Gordon-Evans WJ, Evans RB, Knap KE, et al. Characterization of spatiotemporal gait characteristics in clinically normal dogs and dogs with spinal cord disease. Am J Vet Res 2009;70:1444–9.
5. Hamilton L, Franklin RJ, Jeffery ND. Quantification of deficits in lateral paw positioning after spinal cord injury in dogs. BMC Vet Res 2008;4:47.
6. Olby NJ, Lim JH, Babb K, et al. Gait scoring in dogs with thoracolumbar spinal cord injuries when walking on a treadmill. BMC Vet Res 2014;10:58.
7. Multon S, Franzen R, Poirrier AL, et al. The effect of treadmill training on motor recovery after a partial spinal cord compression-injury in the adult rat. J Neurotrauma 2003;20:699–706.
8. Battistuzzo CR, Callister RJ, Callister R, et al. A systematic review of exercise training to promote locomotor recovery in animal models of spinal cord injury. J Neurotrauma 2012;29:1600–13.
9. Thornton H, Kilbride C. Physical management of abnormal tone and movement. In: Stokes M, editor. Physical management in neurological rehabilitation. 2nd edition. London: Elsevier Mosby; 2004. p. 431–50.
10. Olby N, Levine J, Harris T, et al. Long-term functional outcome of dogs with severe injuries of the thoracolumbar spinal cord: 87 cases (1996–2001). J Am Vet Med Assoc 2003;222:762–9.
11. Kathmann I, Cizinauskas S, Doherr MG, et al. Daily controlled physiotherapy increases survival time in dogs with suspected degenerative myelopathy. J Vet Intern Med 2006;20:927–32.
12. Tofthagen C, Visovsky C, Berry DL. Strength and balance training for adults with peripheral neuropathy and high risk of fall: current evidence and implications for future research. Oncol Nurs Forum 2012;39:E416–24.
13. Fonteyn EM, Heeren A, Engels JJ, et al. Gait adaptability training improves obstacle avoidance and dynamic stability in patients with cerebellar degeneration. Gait Posture 2014;40:247–51.
14. Pollock A, Baer G, Langhorne P, et al. Physiotherapy treatment approaches for the recovery of postural control and lower limb function following stroke: a systematic review. Clin Rehabil 2007;21:395–410.
15. Marsden J, Harris C. Cerebellar ataxia: pathophysiology and rehabilitation. Clin Rehabil 2011;25:195–216.
16. Kwan RL, Cheing GL, Vong SK, et al. Electrophysical therapy for managing diabetic foot ulcers: a systematic review. Int Wound J 2013;10:121–31.
17. Papich MG. Saunders handbook of veterinary drugs: small and large animal. 3rd edition. St Louis (MO): Elsevier Saunders; 2011.
18. Olby N. The pathogenesis and treatment of acute spinal cord injuries in dogs. Vet Clin North Am Small Anim Pract 2010;40:791–807.
19. Furlan AD, Imamura M, Dryden T, et al. Massage for low back pain: an updated systematic review within the framework of the Cochrane Back Review Group. Spine (Phila Pa 1976) 2009;34:1669–84.
20. Field TM. Massage therapy effects. Am Psychol 1998;53:1270–81.
21. Gaynor JS. Acupuncture for management of pain. Vet Clin North Am Small Anim Pract 2000;30:875–84, viii.
22. Zhao ZQ. Neural mechanism underlying acupuncture analgesia. Prog Neurobiol 2008;85:355–75.

23. Levine D, Marcellin-Little DJ, Millis DL, et al. Effects of partial immersion in water on vertical ground reaction forces and weight distribution in dogs. Am J Vet Res 2010;71:1413–6.

24. Schaal CM, Collins L, Ashley C. Cardiorespiratory responses to underwater treadmill running versus land-based treadmill running. Int J Aquat Res Educ 2012;6:35–45.

25. Caetano KS, Frade MA, Minatel DG, et al. Phototherapy improves healing of chronic venous ulcers. Photomed Laser Surg 2009;27:111–8.

26. Dawood MS, Salman SD. Low level diode laser accelerates wound healing. Lasers Med Sci 2013;28:941–5.

27. Esnouf A, Wright PA, Moore JC, et al. Depth of penetration of an 850nm wavelength low level laser in human skin. Acupunct Electrother Res 2007;32:81–6.

28. Malizos KN, Hantes ME, Protopappas V, et al. Low-intensity pulsed ultrasound for bone healing: an overview. Injury 2006;37(Suppl 1):S56–62.

29. Gurgen SG, Sayin O, Cetin F, et al. Transcutaneous electrical nerve stimulation (TENS) accelerates cutaneous wound healing and inhibits pro-inflammatory cytokines. Inflammation 2014;37:775–84.

30. Reed BV. Effect of high voltage pulsed electrical stimulation on microvascular permeability to plasma proteins. A possible mechanism in minimizing edema. Phys Ther 1988;68:491–5.

31. Khadilkar A, Milne S, Brosseau L, et al. Transcutaneous electrical nerve stimulation for the treatment of chronic low back pain: a systematic review. Spine (Phila Pa 1976) 2005;30:2657–66.

Physical Rehabilitation After Total Joint Arthroplasty in Companion Animals

Denis J. Marcellin-Little, DEDV[a],*, Nancy D. Doyle, MPT[b],
Joanna Freeman Pyke, PT, BSc.KINE[c]

KEYWORDS

- Animal rehabilitation • Ambulation assistance • Controlled exercise
- Total hip replacement • Total knee replacement • Total elbow replacement
- Complications

KEY POINTS

- The goal of rehabilitation after total joint arthroplasty (TJA) is the lifelong restoration of a pain-free, functional limb.
- Rehabilitation after TJA includes controlling postoperative pain, minimizing complications, increasing function, restoring range of motion, and increasing strength of the surrounding musculature.
- Rehabilitation after TJA is particularly important in patients at high risk of limb disuse or complication.
- Rehabilitation provides tools for the management of cases experiencing postoperative complications.
- Patients receiving total elbow replacement or total knee replacement typically require much more extensive rehabilitation for optimal functional outcomes than those receiving total hip replacement.

Osteoarthritis (OA) affects many dogs and cats. Even though global statistics on the prevalence of OA in dogs and cats are lacking, statistics from the Orthopedic Foundation for Animals (www.OFFA.org) for the 50 most affected dog breeds indicate that hip dysplasia is present in 21% dogs, based on 430,000 evaluations, and that elbow dysplasia is present in 16% of dogs, based on 180,000 evaluations. When medical management fails to control the pain and disability resulting from OA, total joint

[a] Department of Clinical Sciences, College of Veterinary Medicine, North Carolina State University, NCSU CVM VHC #2563, 1052 William Moore Drive, Raleigh, NC 27607-4065, USA; [b] Gulf Coast Veterinary Specialists, 1111 West Loop South, Houston, TX 77027, USA; [c] Private Practice, 2285 Bristol Circle, Oakville, Ontario L6H 6P8, Canada
* Corresponding author.
E-mail address: djmarcel@ncsu.edu

Vet Clin Small Anim 45 (2015) 145–165
http://dx.doi.org/10.1016/j.cvsm.2014.09.008
0195-5616/15/$ – see front matter © 2015 Elsevier Inc. All rights reserved.

arthroplasties (TJA) can restore lost function and, ultimately, offer pain relief from debilitating OA. However, the impact of OA on the periarticular structures persists during the months that follow surgery, making physical rehabilitation an important aspect of the postoperative management of TJA. Periarticular fibrosis and associated loss of joint motion, muscle atrophy, particularly of type II fibers that provide rapid dynamic support for joint protection, decreased voluntary muscle recruitment, impaired proprioception, osteoporosis, chronic pain, and general physical deconditioning are all associated with chronic arthritic changes in companion animals. Impaired preoperative limb use and mobility in turn compound the postoperative challenges faced during recovery after TJA.

In the weeks that follow surgery, total joint prostheses are vulnerable to complications, requiring skilled care for protection and optimal functional recovery. The rehabilitation environment is ideally suited for patients who are recovering from TJA. Rehabilitation clinicians possess the expertise to safely and effectively restore functional use of patients' operated limbs and ensure maximal recoveries. Rehabilitation clinicians are also uniquely qualified to coordinate client education and communication regarding housing modifications, activity restrictions, and home rehabilitation care for patients recovering from surgery. This article presents rehabilitation considerations for companion animals undergoing total hip replacement (THR), total knee replacement (TKR) and total elbow replacement (TER), postoperative complications and how to mitigate risks, and anticipated patient outcomes. Comparisons are made to physical therapy procedures and expectations after TJA in humans, as the body of clinical research relating to TJA in humans is much larger and richer in scientific evidence than that in companion animals. Because humans and companion animals generally have parallel physiology, for example as it relates to joint motion and bone metabolism, many clinical findings in humans can be judiciously extrapolated to companion animals. However, differences related to joint function must be considered, such as that the elbow is a weight-bearing joint in dogs but not in humans. Most of the companion animal information included in the text refers to TJA for dogs. When information relates to other nonhuman animal species (ie, cats), the species is mentioned specifically in the text.

GOALS OF REHABILITATION AFTER TOTAL JOINT ARTHROPLASTY

The goal of rehabilitation after TJA is the lifelong restoration of a pain-free, functional limb after implantation of the prosthesis. Specific rehabilitation goals include controlling postoperative pain, minimizing complications, increasing function, restoring passive and active range of motion (PROM and AROM), increasing strength of the surrounding musculature, restoring function, and ultimately improving patients' quality of life. Rehabilitation after TJA generally takes 3 months, but adherence to an individualized home exercise program may be warranted for up to 6 months or more, depending on each patient's needs. Most primary soft tissue healing takes place during the first month, with maturation continuing for months beyond that point. The bone-implant interface of cemented implants reaches maximal strength 1 day after surgery, whereas the bone-implant interface of cementless implants relies on bone ingrowth. Most of the bone ingrowth occurs during the first 2 months; afterward, bone remodels slowly during the first year after surgery. Many patients use their operated limb consistently by the end of the first month, walk without lameness by the end of the second month, and can engage in any activity, including training for specific sporting activities by the end of the third month after surgery, depending on patient profile and client goals. These timelines serve to guide rehabilitation and patient activity levels to avoid complications.

A key goal of rehabilitation after TJA is to manage postoperative pain effectively. Many patients undergoing TJA have chronic pain as a result of severe OA. Pain management relies on medications (nonsteroidal anti-inflammatory drugs, opiates, N-methyl-D-aspartate receptor antagonists), on electrophysical modalities and manual therapy, on optimal housing, and on safe transportation (described later in this article). Chronic pain should subside within 3 months after TJA.[1,2] Chronic pain and limb disuse can be present over the long term after TJA but, in the absence of clear complications, they are unusual. If chronic pain or limb disuse persists beyond this normal recovery time period, the presence of an undetected complication should be suspected.

Minimizing the likelihood of complications is another key goal of rehabilitation after TJA. High-risk patients and living situations must be identified, and confinement and therapy must be adapted to mitigate these risk factors. Patients may be at risk because of their profile, including age, size, behavior, training, and conditioning. Older dogs generally have more advanced disease (eg, increased bone loss, chronic joint luxation, severe periarticular fibrosis) and frequently have comorbidities (see next paragraph). They may be more deconditioned, prone to falls due to weakness or balance impairment, and not easy to motivate during recovery. Younger dogs may be unruly, not well trained or socialized, and also prone to falls due to exuberance. Patients that are very large may be at risk of complications because of increased forces placed on implants and implant-bone interfaces, potential clumsiness, and impingement (described later in this article). Fearful or aggressive dogs could be more prone to short-term postoperative complications due to uncontrollable or unexpected bursts and ballistic movements. Patients also may be at risk because of their owners' profiles. Owners may be unwilling to modify the patient's living environment or be unable to care for their companions because of their health, occupation, or motivations.

Comorbidities also increase risk of complications. Classic comorbidities in dogs include concurrent orthopedic diseases that cause dogs to offload and use abnormal gait patterns; examples include OA of the contralateral joint, cranial cruciate ligament injuries, and lumbosacral disease. The obesity epidemic in America extends to our TJA patients, increasing the loads borne by the implanted prostheses. Patients' presurgical lifestyles, preoperative levels of function, strength of associated muscle groups, and endurance have a direct effect on patient outcomes. In dogs, the prevalence of comorbidities and their influence on complications and outcomes of TJA have not been evaluated. Several dog-specific scoring systems evaluating orthopedic disability and mobility[3–5] and a patient-fracture assessment scoring system have been reported.[6] A similar patient-disease index would be beneficial to identify factors that negatively impact the outcome of TJA. In humans, comorbidities in patients undergoing TJA and their influence on functional outcome, implant survival, mortality, and length of hospital stay have been described.[7] Several instruments are used to quantify comorbidity, including comorbidities indices (eg, Charlson index, index of coexistent disease, functional comorbidity index), other health or quality-of-life indices (eg, Charnley index, American Society of Anesthesiologists physical status classification, SF-36), and osteoarthritis indices (eg, Western Ontario and McMaster Osteoarthritis Index [WOMAC], hip osteoarthritis outcomes scale).[8] Other instruments are used to evaluate functional outcomes (eg, lower extremity functional scale [LEFS], timed up and go [TUG test], and range of motion [ROM] measurements [flexion and extension]).[9] Although analogous instruments are not available for assessment of our animal patients with total joint replacement (TJR), it is still important for rehabilitation clinicians to clearly identify and communicate similar functional characteristics of each TJA patient with the surgeon to facilitate detection of potential complications as early as possible in the treatment process. This discussion among all members of the patient's health care team identifies the duration of hospitalization that is safest, the level of nursing care required, and the strategies to minimize complications.

COMPLICATIONS OF TOTAL JOINT ARTHROPLASTY

THR is by far the most common TJA in dogs. Recognized complications of THRs include luxations, fractures, neurapraxia, implant loosening, and infection. The overall complication rate of THR in dogs is approximately 10%.[10]

Luxation of Prosthetic Joints

Luxations are the most common short-term complications of THR, with an incidence ranging from 8% to 12% of THRs.[10,11] Most luxations occur within the first 3 months after surgery. Luxations can result from suboptimal implant positioning; for example, when a cup is too *open* the prosthesis is predisposed to dorsal luxation, and when the cup is too *closed*, the prosthesis is predisposed to ventral luxation.[12] The risk of luxation also increases when the stem is implanted too recessed in the femoral canal or the femoral neck is too short.[13] The stem also can become recessed as a consequence of stem subsidence postoperatively. Luxations also can occur when the cup and stem contact each other during activities of daily living, a phenomenon named *impingement*. In humans, impingement is more likely when the ratio of cup size/prosthetic head size increases.[14] Impingement is most likely a predominant cause of THR luxation in giant-breed dogs, which seemingly are at increased risk (**Fig. 1**).[13] Most femoral heads have diameters ranging from 16 to 18 mm, but one manufacturer (BioMedtrix, Boonton, NJ, USA) recently introduced a larger femoral head measuring 22 mm to decrease the risk of impingement in giant-breed dogs. Luxations can result from impingement of the femur and ischium or from a thick, fibrous joint capsule, sometimes seen in older German shepherd dogs and other breeds.[10] In all cases in which luxations occur due to suboptimal implant positioning, surgical revisions are indicated for successful reduction and prevention of recurrence.

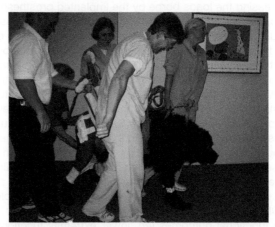

Fig. 1. A 4-year-old neutered male Newfoundland weighing 104 kg (230 lb) is learning to walk on the day after a surgery that reduced a ventral luxation of a total hip implant placed 2 years earlier. The dog is controlled and supported by a check harness and 2 slings. Hobbles made of adhesive tape prevent excessive abduction of the operated limb. One week later, the dog could walk independently without support. The pelvic limbs were hobbled for 5 months. The hip did not re-luxate afterward.

Pelvic limb amputees undergoing THR on the remaining pelvic limb also are at increased risk of luxation because they stand and walk with their pelvis tilted toward the side of amputation, placing the THR in relative adduction and decreasing dorsal coverage of the femoral head.[15] The posture of these patients may be improved with exercise.

Traumatic luxations can occur when patients fall into a splayed posture (ventral luxation) or onto the hip (dorsal luxation), underscoring the need for supported ambulation and measures to prevent slips or losses of balance. Patients with ventral hip luxations resulting from excessive limb abduction (eg, slipping and *doing the splits*) can be managed with closed reduction and placement of hobbles that limit abduction (see **Fig. 1**), provided that the luxation is not the result of impingement of the femoral neck on the acetabular cup. Joints with impingement are likely to re-luxate during normal activities and require surgical repositioning of the implants for successful outcomes. Dorsal luxations also may be treated with closed reduction and temporary immobilization with an Ehmer sling or they may require surgical revision. Several investigators proposed that nontraumatic luxations occurring 6 weeks to 4 months after surgery may be the consequence of inadequate recovery of muscle support and periarticular soft tissue healing.[12,16] Although not yet validated through research, rehabilitation of patients identified to be at increased risk of luxation could potentially decrease the occurrence of luxation in this population.

Femoral Fracture

Femoral fractures are a common complication of THR in dogs, occurring both intraoperatively and postoperatively at rates ranging from 2% to 8%.[10,17] A femur could be at risk of fracture because of thin cortices. The femoral fractures that occur during surgery are often stabilized with cerclage wires placed around the femoral shaft. After appropriate cerclage placement, prosthetic stems resist subsidence as much as stems placed in nonfractured femurs, thus not placing the patient at an increased risk of luxation from subsidence.[18] Postoperatively, fractures can occur when undetected surgically induced fissures propagate, when excessive loading occurs before adequate cortical hypertrophy has developed, or as a result of trauma. These fractures usually necessitate surgical stabilization. The rehabilitation plan for patients with THRs and fractures should include a focus on maintaining length/flexibility of the quadriceps and hamstrings due to the impact that fractures and fixation have on these muscles.

Sciatic Neurapraxia

Sciatic nerve neurapraxia is an infrequent complication of THR, occurring in 1.6% to 1.9% of patients.[19,20] Sciatic neurapraxia can occur after THR due to compression of the nerve intraoperatively, in the vicinity of the ischiatic spine during gluteal retraction or between the caudal joint capsule and the ischiatic tuberosity. Patients with sciatic nerve palsy have an abnormal gait. They have impaired active stifle and tarsal flexion, scuff or knuckle their paws, and use increased hip flexion to advance the limb and clear the ground when walking. Sciatic nerve neurapraxia is generally transient, lasting for a few weeks to a few months, but can be permanent. Geriatric dogs and those undergoing longer surgeries have increased risk of postoperative sciatic neurapraxia.[20]

Infection

Infection can occur after THR.[10] Presentation may be acute, with limb swelling and hyperthermia, or chronic (low-grade infection) without swelling or systemic signs. Most THR infections are low-grade infections developing weeks to months after surgery, most often from bacteria introduced at the time of surgery or possibly as the result of hematogenous infection. Infection should be suspected in patients that exhibit progressively poorer limb use (because of persistent pain) after an initially uneventful recovery in the absence of radiographic evidence of fracture or loosening. Infection can be confirmed if specific bone changes are visible on radiographs and a bacterial culture of the joint space or regional tissues is positive. Infection is often a devastating complication because antibiotic therapy is unlikely to sterilize the bone-implant interface. Explantation of the THR prosthesis may be required, leaving the patient with what is essentially a femoral head ostectomy. These patients require extensive rehabilitation and more aggressive pain management to restore functional use of the limb.

Failure of Fixation

Stems or cups used in THR can be loose either because of lack of bone ingrowth into cementless implants or because of aseptic loosening over time. The acetabular cup may at increased risk of failure of fixation because of a defect to the medial acetabular wall (*protrusio*) or dorsal acetabular rim. The bone ingrowth that occurs in the first 6 to 8 weeks after surgery is critical to long-term prosthesis stability. Excessive activity during this time period causes a disruption of the healing due to the development of a fibrous membrane between the implant and the bone, described as fibrous ingrowth. Loose implants generate an inflammatory response in the bone (visible on radiographs) that progresses slowly over time. Like low-grade infections, their presence leads to poor limb use and progressive loss of muscle mass.

Complications of Total Knee Replacement (TKR) and Total Elbow Replacement (TER)

The complications of other total joints are similar to the complications of THR. After TKR, collateral ligament damage (and secondary stifle subluxation), infection, fractures, and luxation have been encountered.[21] The medial or lateral collateral ligaments can be damaged during surgery, usually during the proximal tibial osteotomy, or can rupture after surgery, particularly if early exuberant activity is permitted, leading to joint instability.[22] Ruptured ligaments must be repaired and protected for several weeks after surgery. Custom orthoses can effectively shield the stifle from varus or valgus forces to facilitate healing, but require significant owner compliance for effective use. Strengthening of the hip stabilizers during recovery ensures the limb is kept in normal alignment and avoids postures that place the stifle under increased varus or valgus loads. Similarly, collateral ligament instability, infection, and fractures can occur after TER.[23] Because osteotomies of the medial or the lateral epicondyle may be performed during implantation (based on the implant systems used), collateral ligament instability may result from avulsion of an epicondylar osteotomy site or epicondylar screw loosening. Ulnar fractures adjacent to the trochlear notch have been reported after TER.[23] Limb amputation may be required for resolution of infection because TERs and TKRs do not have the option of explantation because unarticulated elbow or stifle joints are completely dysfunctional.

MANAGEMENT AFTER TOTAL JOINT ARTHROPLASTY
Hospitalization and Aftercare

Patients recovering from TJA are most often managed as inpatients in the early postoperative period. Inpatient management allows the dogs to be handled by a limited number of caregivers who are familiar with the specific needs related to each patient's personality, pain levels, mobility, and risk profile. These needs are described in the following text. Inpatient management can last a few days for low-risk patients and can last several weeks for high-risk patients or in instances in which the owners are unwilling or unable to care for their pet during recovery.

After discharge from the hospital, patients recovering from TJA are either treated as rehabilitation outpatients or are solely managed at home. Some THR patients are treated at home because transportation to and from the rehabilitation facility presents risks associated with getting in and out of motor vehicles, walking on slippery clinic flooring, and encountering uncontrolled environmental challenges, such as other patients at the facility. Risks are minimized when dogs are walked at a slow, controlled speed using appropriate equipment, thus increasing their safe, functional mobility in the early days after surgery. A chest harness (Step In Harness TEC; Canine Equipment, Vancouver, Canada) provides more control than a collar and allows weight-bearing support of the forelimbs after TER. A thin support sling (**Fig. 2**) should be used to provide additional weight-bearing support of the pelvic limbs for dogs needing ambulation assistance and prevent falls. Commercial support systems (Help'Em Up; Blue Dog Designs, Denver, CO, USA) also can be used. Even if donning and doffing them require manipulation, dogs usually tolerate harnesses well and can wear them all day. Owners remove harnesses at night and inspect the skin for hair loss, redness, and abrasions. Harnesses also are removed and cleaned when soiled (eg, by urine or feces). These support measures also should be used at home when dogs are taken outside to relieve themselves and during the brief periods of exercise permitted in

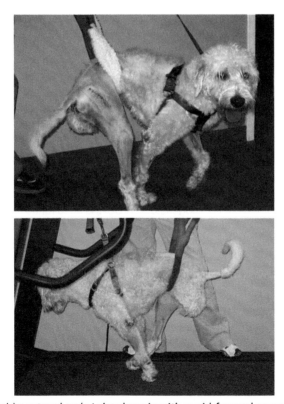

Fig. 2. A 1-year-old neutered male Labrador mix with a mid-femoral amputation is learning to walk the day after a contralateral THR done to manage a chronic untreated acetabular fracture. The dog is uncoordinated. He is supported with a chest harness and a sling at all times. Gait training includes slow walks (*top*) and walking on a treadmill, 10 days after surgery (*bottom*).

the early postoperative period. A leash measuring less than 1 m (approximately 3 feet) should be used. Support slings and harness supporting the abdomen and pelvic limbs enhance control of the patient and decrease the likelihood of falls. Assistance during transitions also should be provided when needed (eg, sit to stand, controlled lowering to sit or lie down).

Care is needed for safe transport. Lighter dogs can be securely lifted in and out of motor vehicles. Heavy dogs can use ramps to get in and out of motor vehicles with the support and protection of slings. Ramps should be rigid and stable and long enough to create a gradual slope. Ramps are more manageable for owners to set up and disassemble when they are telescoping (Deluxe XL Telescoping Pet Ramp; Solvit, Arlington, TX, USA) or can be folded (UltraLite Bi-fold Pet Ramp; Solvit) or rolled (Ramp4Paws, Potomac, MD, USA). In cars or trucks, dogs should be allowed to rest on flat surfaces, ideally secured through their harness/seatbelt or accompanied by a second attendant to ensure they do not attempt to move about while the vehicle is in motion. Tight spaces and gaps present risks of limb entrapment and injury. Smaller dogs are safest traveling in crates and also can be transported in the facility while in this confinement.

At home, dogs should be confined to a large exercise pen or small single room when unsupervised. The patient should feel comfortable in that room and not exhibit undue stress. Room modifications should include secure footing (carpeting or rugs), a dog bed at floor level, and removal of furniture that the dog may attempt to climb on (ie, couches and chairs). The room should be away from windows or doors that may trigger explosive responses (eg, the postal carrier stops by or a guest knocks on the door). When directly supervised, patients can be kept in larger rooms, provided they have acceptable mobility and the same precautions are taken. Stairs pose specific challenges, particularly when they cannot be avoided (eg, the owner lives in an apartment on an upper level or has a multilevel home with living spaces upstairs). Strategies should be developed with the owner to use the aforementioned support devices, enlisting help of neighbors or family members if needed (in the acute phases of recovery for larger dogs), or make temporary alternative living arrangements. As long as these safeguards are in place, stairs can be negotiated as soon as patients return home.

Owners often request oral medications for active, boisterous patients that may help keep them calm during confinement and exercise restriction after TJA. Acepromazine maleate (Boehringer Ingelheim, Ridgefield, CT, USA) is used for its sedative properties but is rarely used in the long term because its safety profile is considered suboptimal. Side effects include hypotension, excessive or prolonged sedation, ataxia, lowered seizure threshold, and dysphoria, all of which may increase the risk for falls and injury. Trazodone hydrochloride (Desyrel; Bristol-Myers Squibb, New York City, NY, USA), a serotonin antagonist and reuptake inhibitor, has been given to dogs after orthopedic surgery and appears to have acceptable safety.[24] In an open trial, most owners (32 of 36, 89%) reported that trazodone improved confinement tolerance moderately or extremely.[25] Current research assessing the efficacy of trazodone after THR suggests that some dogs may be rated as calmer even when owners give placebo (Dr BL Sherman, North Carolina State University, personal communication, 2014). The belief of giving a medication to improve confinement tolerance might lead to behavior modification by owners that would promote calmness. To help ease patient "boredom" and restlessness, gentle play (eg, gentle tug-of-war) is safe; instruction in simple tricks and commands also serves as fun interactive time with the owner and provides mental stimulation for patients during convalescence. Puzzle toys that dogs manipulate to access food also may be provided for supervised distractions. Protected movement, albeit controlled, should be encouraged.

Wound Management

Wound healing after TJA is important. There is no report of skin infection progressing to implant infection in companion animals, to our knowledge. Nevertheless, wound infections can cause dehiscence of the surgical incision and could lead to deep tissue infections (as they do in humans). Wound management includes covering the incision with an adhesive bandage until the incision is sealed, approximately 5 days after surgery, or until suture removal 10 to 14 days after surgery. If the wound is not covered, disinfecting the skin incision periodically (0.05% chlorhexidine diacetate, Nolvasan; Zoetis, Florham Park, NJ, USA) or placing a thin layer of triple antibiotic ointment could be beneficial. Elizabethan collars or alternative donut-style collars may be used in dogs showing signs of self-mutilation. Dogs generally dislike Elizabethan collars and may struggle to remove them, potentially putting the procedure at risk for complications.

REHABILITATION METHODS AFTER TOTAL JOINT ARTHROPLASTY

Electrophysical modalities, manual therapies, and therapeutic exercises are used for the rehabilitation of patients undergoing TJA. Cryotherapy (cold packs) begins immediately postoperatively and continues through the inflammatory phase to decrease postoperative pain and swelling. Cryotherapy is safe, well tolerated, and technically simple. Cold packs can be used several times daily for approximately 10 to 15 minutes, until the skin is cold to the touch. In humans, cryotherapy decreases blood loss after TJA in general (but not after THR), provides pain relief on the day after surgery (but not on day 1 or 3) and improves quadriceps muscle activation after TKR.[26,27] Nontoxic gel packs should be used and patients should be carefully monitored throughout administration to ensure the packs are not chewed or ingested.

Manual therapy plays an important role in recovery for many patients after TJA, particularly those with ROM restrictions. In humans, restoration of flexion and extension ROM is imperative after TKR surgery and is generally pursued with physical therapy interventions beginning as soon as the first day after surgery. Specific motion restrictions in human patients with THR are more commonly addressed in physiotherapy practices 6 weeks after surgery, once the surgeon lifts the protective motion restrictions. Massage may be used to decrease pain and edema and to promote motion between tissue planes. In humans, back massage reportedly decreases pain after THR and TKR.[28] Passive ROM completed in the early phases of recovery helps avoid postoperative stiffness, improve comfort, and begin restoration of joint motion. In humans, the use of a continuous passive motion machine (CPM) decreases length of stay after TJA because of improved active joint motion but its long-term benefits are unclear.[29] Active, active assisted, and passive ROM exercises are an alternative to CPM and are implemented immediately after surgery. These exercises continue via a home exercise program after discharge from active physiotherapy and should continue up to 12 weeks after surgery or until specific goals are reached.

In dogs, the same goals and interventions apply. Therefore, early interventions to increase ROM and influence the organization of scar tissue are key to regaining lost motion and decreasing pain (**Fig. 3**). If early intervention is not provided, unnecessary stiffness sets in and, in turn, is harder to reverse. In some human patients, manipulation under anesthesia is warranted if exuberant adhesions or fibrosis preclude restoration of ROM at an expected rate postoperatively. Preventing complications and setting a path for recovery based on proven techniques delivered by trained therapists is paramount. Heat therapy may be combined with ROM and passive stretching techniques to improve the pliability of the target tissues, but this should not be done until

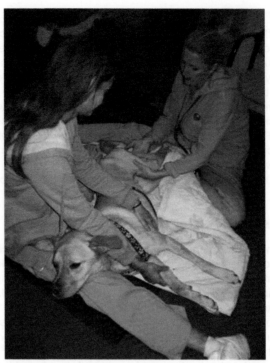

Fig. 3. A patient with THR is held in lateral recumbency for a massage and stretching session a few days after surgery. The hip region lacked extension, and a severe pain response was present on extension.

the active, acute inflammation has subsided. More advanced stretching (particularly joint flexion, as in the case of TKR) can also be performed during specific active therapeutic exercises that stimulate the patient to move the affected joint through the targeted ROM. For example, when the patient sits, the hip and stifle are normally placed in flexion. If the patient lacks full flexion, the patient may compensate by sitting "side swept" (both limbs positioned to one side via spinal rotation) or in a "lazy sit" (abducting the affected limb or sitting back on the ischii to position the limb cranially). Modifications can be made to accommodate the restrictions and allow the patient to maximally flex and stretch, such as cuing the dog to sit on the handler's leg or platform or minimally abducting the affected limb (**Fig. 4**). Loss of extension ROM can be more functionally debilitating and interfere with proper limb use and weight bearing than loss of flexion ROM. If full extension is not restored, then the loss of ROM at end range may mimic a leg length discrepancy and ultimately impair weight bearing of the affected limb. Exercises that cue active stifle extension include sit to stands, uphill walking, walking backward, and reaching for a treat with the forelimbs elevated (**Fig. 5**). Ideally, both flexion and extension ROM should be restored to normal limits after TJR to provide the patient the best functional outcome.

SPECIFIC REHABILITATION PROGRAMS FOR DOGS UNDERGOING TOTAL JOINT ARTHROPLASTY

Completion of therapeutic exercises while hospitalized and at home optimizes limb use after TJA in humans and companion animals. Large dogs and high-risk patients

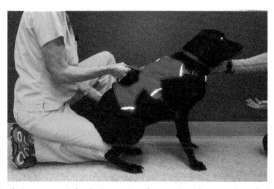

Fig. 4. A patient is doing a modified sit to stand exercise that is aimed at strengthening his pelvic limbs and stretching his hip and stifle in flexion. The dog sits on the handler's knee. That elevated position requires less hip and knee flexion. A harness provides control and any needed assistance.

may need training to learn to get up and walk (see **Fig. 1**). Patients with TKR and TER need exercise to initiate and promote use of their operated limbs, particularly if they had very limited use of the limbs preoperatively. All patients with TJR benefit from increased strength (strengthening their operated limb). In the long term, patients with TJR should remain active and strong through exercise. This increased strength and conditioning improves the patient's quality of life and thus, the owners' satisfaction with the surgical outcome. Specific therapeutic exercises for THR, TKR, and TER are described in the following sections.

Total Hip Replacement

Dog are most often hospitalized for 1 to 3 days after THR. A middle-age large-breed dog with good mobility and good limb use can safely be discharged the day after surgery if pain is controlled on oral and patch analgesics. Hospitalization is prolonged when the perceived risk of complication is higher, when postoperative limb use is

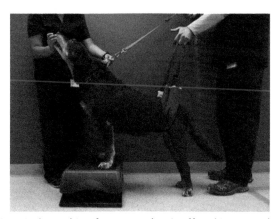

Fig. 5. A patient is actively reaching for a treat that is offered in a way that promotes pushing with his pelvic limbs into stifle and hip extension. The sling under his belly (The Soft Quick Lift, Four Flags Over Aspen, St Clair, MN, USA), is used to protect against falls and to maintain control. This exercise can be modulated in difficulty by varying the height of the step or by progressing to an unsteady "step," such as a balance disc or Physioroll.

poor, or when pain levels necessitate intensive medical management. Cold therapy may be applied 2 or 3 times a day to the operated area during the hospitalization period. Patients should be kept in a calm environment and in an enclosure large enough to allow the patient to comfortably reposition but small enough to avoid running or jumping. The enclosure should have nonslip flooring (**Fig. 6**). Once home, dogs should be confined as previously described. A belly or pelvic limb sling should be used until dogs are *confidently* using their operated limb. Most often, a sling becomes unnecessary 2 to 3 weeks after surgery and the dog can then be controlled solely with a chest harness or collar and leash. Once the dog is walking confidently, typically 2 to 3 weeks after surgery, leash walks can increase progressively. Subjectively, most patients can walk for 5 minutes without lameness by the end of the first month after surgery, 15 minutes by the end of the second month, and 30 minutes by the end of the third month. Patients are palpated and radiographs are made 3 months after surgery. More strenuous activities can resume progressively and preferably under the direction of a skilled rehabilitation clinician or trainer.

Several retrospective and a few prospective studies of canine THR have been published.[10] They included little information regarding postoperative rehabilitation beyond initial supportive care and progressive leash walks. In a long-term prospective clinical trial in which physical rehabilitation was limited to walking dogs on a leash to void during the first 2 months after surgery and increasing the length of leash walks during weeks 9 to 12, hip PROM was normal in 29 (94%) of 31 dogs that were free of complications 5 years after surgery.[11] Hip extension was decreased in 3 dogs with long-term implant luxation and in 1 dog with a femoral osteosarcoma. In the same study, thigh girth was equal or larger to the opposite thigh in all dogs that were complication-free. To our knowledge, there are no published reports describing dogs that did not achieve proper limb function after THR, provided that the hips were free of implant malposition, infection, fracture, or failure of fracture fixation. Functionally, dogs undergoing routine THR have normal limb use 3 months after surgery.[2] This suggests that specific rehabilitation programs or long hospitalization periods are probably not necessary for the success of uncomplicated THRs but they may be considered in patients with limited hip joint motion because of tissue tightness. For example, some patients with dorsal femoral displacement for extended periods of time before surgery have tight periarticular muscles and other soft tissues after joint

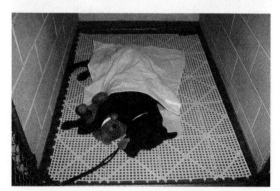

Fig. 6. A patient with THR is waking up from anesthesia in a small run with nonskid flooring. Once body temperature returns to normal, the heating blanket and covers will be removed to avoid tripping the patient. The sides and door of the run are high to dissuade the dog from jumping or standing on his rear limbs to peer over the sides or attempt to get out.

reduction during surgery, including external rotators, gluteal muscles, and rectus femoris. These tight muscles interfere with comfortable locomotion and may result in a characteristic "hockey stick" posture of hip external rotation and abduction, positioning the paw laterally. Subjectively, periarticular restrictions due to chronic OA typically result in decreased hip extension, internal rotation, and abduction. Of these movement planes, extension most impacts the patient's mobility and function. Human patients with THR work to restore lost hip flexion, extension, internal and external rotation lost during the 12 weeks of contraindicated movements placed on them. Hip abduction weakness is one of the most measurable impairments in human patients with THR, but is likely of lesser importance in dogs, considering their quadrupedal gait.

Dogs with limited hip extension will benefit from a stretching program. When the loss of hip extension is severe, moist heat and manual stretching techniques are used. Extension uses a spinning motion of the femoral head on the acetabulum and thus tightens the joint capsule at end ranges. This is a safe direction for stretching with regard to very limited possibility for luxating the hip with overzealous motion, but care must be exercised to not cause patient pain with this stretch. Following the stretching session, active hip extension exercises should be performed to retrain the patient to use the increased ROM. When the loss of hip extension is modest and the patient's limb use is acceptable, manual stretching may not be critical. Some patients are not receptive to stretching techniques and owners cannot safely perform stretching at home. For both of these populations, targeted therapeutic exercises alone can be used instead to gain hip extension for a more normal gait pattern and better function. Walking up a gentle incline, stepping up a single step or a series of steps with adequate traction, and stepping over objects all place the trailing limb in increased hip extension (**Fig. 7**).

Dogs experiencing complications following THR have additional rehabilitation needs. Following the acute management of a luxation (with reduction/hobbles and/or surgical revision), targeted strengthening of the appropriate muscle groups provides improved dynamic joint support to help prevent a recurrence. Dogs that experienced a dorsal luxation need additional strengthening of the muscles lying on the dorsal aspect of the hip. Suggested exercises include 3-legged standing (lifting the

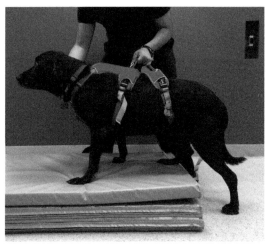

Fig. 7. A patient is doing a *step up* exercise in which the dog repeatedly steps up on a mat, promoting extension in the operated left hip. A harness (Web Master Harness, Ruffwear, Bend, OR, USA) is used to provide support against falling and to control speed.

unaffected pelvic limb and cuing the dog to shift weight onto the operative limb while maintaining a level pelvis), balancing on a soft or unsteady surface (commercial balance discs or an air mattress), walking perpendicular to an incline with the operative limb "downhill," and the previously mentioned hip extension exercises. Dogs experiencing a ventral luxation require strengthening of the adductors. Suggested exercises include resisted TheraBand exercise (TheraBand, Akron, OH, USA) while walking on a treadmill or alongside the handler (pull the hip into abduction with the band wrapped around the thigh to stimulate a contraction of the adductors), walking sideways, or walking perpendicular to an incline with the operative limb "uphill." Underwater treadmill walking also can effectively and safely target the desired muscle group in both cases, particularly in the earlier phases of recovery. Proprioceptive retraining also should be used to improve body awareness and coordination for decreased risk of future falls.

Patients with sciatic neurapraxia typically present with knuckling and weakness of the muscles in the sciatic distribution, including the hamstrings and crus musculature. Dogs exhibiting deficits due to sciatic neurapraxia after THR need rehabilitation for days to months, depending on the severity of the deficits.[20] Rehabilitation focuses on minimizing hip complications due to decreased active muscular stabilization and protection (eg, luxation), avoiding skin abrasions resulting from scuffing or knuckling, decreasing the loss of muscle mass in muscles innervated by branches of the sciatic nerve, and strengthening the affected muscle groups. Neuromuscular electrical stimulation can be used to elicit muscle contractions of the affected muscles to attenuate atrophy but is not universally well accepted by patients, particularly when sensation is intact. If active hock extension is absent for weight bearing, the hock can be stabilized by an orthosis during therapeutic exercises (**Fig. 8**). Once hock extension improves, the dog can exercise without an orthosis. To avoid abrasions, affected dogs should avoid walking on abrasive surfaces and metacarpals and toes should be protected by a thin bootie or bandage. If the patient frequently knuckles, bootie systems with support straps that pull the hock into flexion and the digits into extension (TheraPaw, Lebanon, NJ, USA) can be used during ambulation and therapeutic exercise sessions to create more normal posture for functional limb use while simultaneously protecting the skin from abrasions. In dogs with weak hock flexion, an exercise band or rubber traction band (Anti-Knuckling Device; Canine Mobility, Seattle, WA, USA or Biko Mobility, Raleigh, NC, USA) can be used to facilitate more normal flexion ROM during exercise. Exercises to strengthen hock flexion include stepping over progressively taller objects, such as segments of PVC pipe, walking in water at the height of the hock, and elicitation of a flexor withdraw reflex by pinching the digits. Most dogs fully recover from sciatic neurapraxia.[20]

Total Knee Replacement

There are few studies reporting the results of TKR in dogs. In 2 experimental studies, TKR was performed in purpose-bred dogs that did not undergo any physical rehabilitation in the postoperative period.[22,30] In one of these, operated stifles lost approximately 32° of ROM excursion in the long term compared with opposite normal stifles (~80° vs ~112°), even though the prostheses were implanted into normal, healthy stifles without preoperative osteoarthritic changes.[22]

The rehabilitation protocol of a prospective clinical study in 6 clinical patients undergoing TKR has been reported.[21] The ROM of the operated knee and thigh girth around the joint line were recorded preoperatively and immediately after surgery for comparison. An ice pack was then applied to the cranial, medial, and lateral aspects of the stifle for 12 minutes. Passive ROM followed by cold pack application was

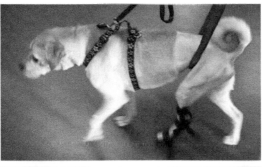

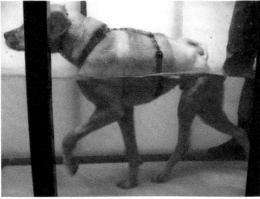

Fig. 8. A patient with THR with sciatic neurapraxia is walking with an orthosis on his left pelvic limb (*top*). The dog can exercise without scuffing or knuckling in an underwater treadmill (*bottom*). Atrophy of the thigh muscles is visible.

repeated 3 times daily while the dog was hospitalized (duration of hospitalization was not specified). After discharge, owners were provided with written and verbal instructions to complete the following sequential activities: short, slow leash walks to stimulate use of the operated limb when outside to void, PROM flexion and extension of the joint as tolerated, and cold pack application for 12 minutes. Two weeks postoperatively, the dogs returned for suture removal and examination by the surgeon and physical therapist. At that time, outpatient rehabilitation was begun and focused on underwater treadmill walking for gait retraining and strengthening, manual therapies to restore stifle PROM and to address concurrent compensatory changes in other joints, and cold packs after exercise to control inflammation. Low-level LASER also could be safely implemented to the stifle to decrease pain and inflammation of the soft tissues and to support the cascade of cellular healing that occurs. Therapy was typically continued 2 to 3 times per week. Four weeks postoperatively, active home exercises were started to target each patient's individual needs, including AROM, strengthening, proprioceptive retraining, and functional retraining. Joint PROM, kinematic gait analysis using a force plate, and limb girth of affected and contralateral limbs were assessed 2 weeks, 6 weeks, 3 months, 6 months, and 12 months after surgery. Stifle joint motion improved within 3 months and remained within normal limits afterward. Mean stifle flexion was 42° before surgery and 37° 1 year after surgery. Mean stifle extension was 143° before surgery and 152° 1 year after surgery. Kinetic gait variables (eg, peak vertical force [PVF], vertical impulse) did not differ statistically after 3 months but were larger after 6 months, indicating that recovery after TKR in dogs is much slower than after THR and more closely mirrors the recovery exhibited by human patients with TKR. One year after TKR, kinetic variables did not equal the contralateral limb if it was normal (PVF improved from 53% before surgery to 82% 1 year after surgery) but exceeded the contralateral limb when OA was present. However, favorable functional improvements and high client satisfaction with outcomes were reported. These outcomes are consistent with the improvements expected after a human TKR.

Although purpose-bred dogs with normal stifle joint may independently restore appropriate limb use after TKR, clinical patients with severe preexisting joint disease always need rehabilitation to normalize limb use and gait mechanics, address comorbidities, and restore lost strength and conditioning, preferably with a focus on function. Patients are frequently non–weight bearing before surgery and have extensive periarticular changes, including fibrosis and weakness that require skilled intervention to elicit positive changes and aid recovery after surgery (**Fig. 9**).

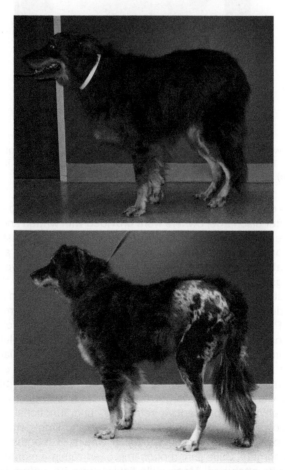

Fig. 9. An 8-year-old spayed female Australian shepherd mix is seen before (*top*) and 2 weeks after TKR (*bottom*). Before surgery, the stifles are held in excessive flexion and the dog is shifting weight forward. After surgery, the dog's posture and weight distribution are improved.

Total Elbow Replacement

Several clinical studies describe the outcome of TER.[23] In the initial study describing implantation of the Iowa State University TER system, experimental dogs were immobilized for 2 weeks by use of a spica splint and therapeutic exercises were initiated 6 weeks after surgery.[23] In the clinical study of the Iowa State University TER system, dogs were bandaged for 1 to 3 days, rested for 2 weeks in a kennel, then leash walked for 15 minutes twice daily, and swum for 15 minutes 3 times per week for 4 weeks. The dogs continued the leash walks for 6 additional weeks. The dogs had unrestricted activity after 12 weeks.[31] In a more recent report, dogs receiving TATE prostheses (BioMedtrix, Boonton, NJ, USA) were protected with a soft, padded bandage for a few days. Dogs were typically discharged 2 days after surgery with instructions to perform regular PROM and massage and to limit exercise for 4 to 6 weeks.[23] Implant stability was confirmed clinically and radiographically 6 weeks after surgery. With confirmation of stability, active therapeutic exercises were begun, including underwater treadmill walks, swimming, and walking across and squatting under Cavaletti rails. PVFs after TER continued to improve over a 12-month period, indicating that functional recovery after TER is a very lengthy process, much slower than recovery after THR and potentially slower than recovery after TKR. Just like patients with TKR, all patients with TER need rehabilitation for maximal recovery (**Fig. 10**).

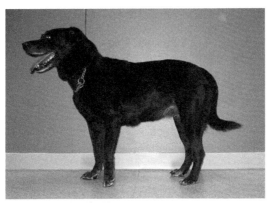

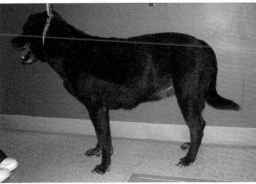

Fig. 10. A 10-year-old spayed female Labrador retriever with severe OA of the left elbow joint is seen before (*top*) and 6 weeks after TER (*bottom*). Before surgery, the dog is non–weight bearing on the left forelimb. After surgery, the dog's use of the operated limb is improved.

Most current TER systems for dogs are bicompartmental; they include a humero-radial and humero-ulnar joint but do not include a radio-ulnar joint.[32] These TERs eliminate radio-ulnar motion. Functionally, the antebrachium is fixed in a pronated position, eliminating supination. The rotational demands placed on the shoulder are increased to compensate for the lack of supination. This may predispose to overuse injuries (bicipital tenosynovitis, medial glenohumeral ligament sprain). Therapy after TER should strengthen the stabilizing rotator cuff muscles surrounding the shoulder joint.

Rehabilitation After Total Joint Arthroplasty in Cats

THR has been performed in cats.[33] TKR also has been performed in a few cats.[34] In a recent report describing THR in 3 cats,[33] patients were discharged the day after surgery and the owners were instructed to prevent jumping and unsupervised activity; if necessary, confinement to a cage for 6 weeks afterward was recommended. Rehabilitation exercises were not recommended. Excellent functional outcomes, defined as being able to sit, stand, walk normally, and jump comfortably without the use of any analgesic medications, were reported in all 3 cats at the final reevaluation (mean follow-up, 11 months).

The goals of rehabilitation after TJA are similar in cats and dogs: pain control, restoration of joint motion and strength, and return to maximal function. Cats present unique challenges during recovery after TJA. Cats tend to be more independent and harder to motivate than dogs, but most can successfully undergo rehabilitation programs.[35,36] Cats have the tendency to jump and climb and should avoid these activities during recovery. Home modifications to prevent jumping during early convalescence are even more important for cats than dogs. Cats can be housed in a large cage during that period. Cats' tolerance of stretches is more variable than dogs' so owner safety must be kept in mind. Home exercise programs are usually less structured than for dogs and involve setting up "equipment" for the cat to encounter in the course of the day (eg, Cavaletti rails across hallways, ramps or steps to access favorite perches). In patients with THR and femoral head ostectomy, strengthening of hip extensor muscles (gluteal and hamstring muscles) is important for jumping. Active exercises under controlled condition (eg, batting a toy with the forelimbs, or following a LASER pointer light on nonslip surfaces) are most engaging to cats and can provide strengthening of the hip extensors through stimulation of antigravity positioning into progressive hip extension. The report of cat THR suggested that it is safe for cats to resume normal activity after 6 weeks of confinement.[33]

ASSESSING PATIENT PROGRESS AND OUTCOMES

Patient progress after TJA guides the rehabilitation. Although patients progress at individual rates, previous sections of this article have given anticipated timelines for the reaching of recovery milestones. These milestones include adequate PROM, AROM, acceptable limb use during activities of daily living, return of muscle mass, and return to full function. With very few exceptions, AROM and limb use start within a few days after THR but return is much slower after TKR and TER. If use of the surgical limb is not seen at the 2-week reevaluation, the patient should be assessed for the previously discussed complications that can occur. Once mechanical and biological causes of disuse are ruled out, pain must be managed effectively using medications and non-pharmaceutical strategies (eg, ice, massage, PROM, transcutaneous electrical nerve stimulation, low-level LASER). When successful pain management results in limb use, active rehabilitation can begin. As with most conditions, the recovery from TJA is not completely linear, but significant declines are not anticipated. If at any time the patient exhibits a decline in function or a loss of the gains previously attained, that should be seen as a "red flag" and investigation for a cause should commence.

Multiple objective measures are used to evaluate the clinical, functional, and economic impacts of TJA in humans. Functional scores include knee society scores, Harris hip score, TUG test, WOMAC, SF-12 and SF-36, 6-Minute Walk Test, and others.[8,37] In companion animals, objective clinical assessments include zonal radiographic analysis, goniometric measures of joint ROM, muscle mass (clinically determined via circumferential limb measures using a tape measure and compared with the contralateral limb), kinetic assessment using a force plate or pressure sensitive walkway, and kinematic analysis. Descriptive measures of functional abilities and limb usage, such as transfers to/from the ground and stair usage, and owner reports of functional changes at home (eg, ability to get on and off furniture, navigate the doggy door, posture to void, including standing on an operative limb while hiking the contralateral one) also serve as meaningful outcome assessments. Although several functional scales have been proposed,[3,5] validated joint scores or functional scores have not been used to assess the outcomes of TJA in companion animals.

Owners are most often satisfied with clinical and functional outcomes of TJA. THR is more commonly performed than TKR, TER, and other total joints (eg, custom TJR). THR appears to have the highest success rate of all TJA, ranging from 80% to 96%, based on evaluation criteria and methods and on length of follow-up.[10] Owners' expectations for high levels of function are consistently met, with our patients routinely returning to active, sporting lives. The prosthesis is expected to last the lifetime of the patient, even when implanted at a young age. Comparatively, if a salvage procedure, such as a femoral head ostectomy, is elected, expectations are modulated to functional, but not normal, limb use with relative patient comfort that may necessitate intermittent use of pain medications, as the biomechanics of the joint have been disrupted and full limb use is rarely restored.

Owner expectations for their dog's recovery after TER or TKR also remain high but are more modest. Case selection for these implants focuses on dogs with profound joint dysfunction and end-stage joint disease where other surgical options would have limited or no benefits (eg, arthroscopy, sliding humeral osteotomy, tibial plateau leveling osteotomy or tibial tuberosity advancement). As such, most of these patients are older and less active. Restoration of a functional limb improves quality of life, alleviates pain, and helps prevent overuse injuries in the other limbs. Published outcomes indicate these goals are consistently met following TER and TKR.[21,23,31] Although a return to normal life for some patients encompasses higher-level activities, such as chasing a flying disc and ball play, many patients return to being "couch potatoes" and family members, with fewer physical demands. As use of these implants expands and prosthetic design advances, case selection also may grow to encompass increasingly young, active dogs with higher physical demands and expectations. The role of rehabilitation in successfully meeting these expectations will remain critical.

In conclusion, patients with TJA have varying needs related to rehabilitation. Rehabilitation should be used in all dogs to identify high-risk patients and to minimize the likelihood of postoperative complications. Many patients undergoing THR recover uneventfully without needing long-term physiotherapy. All patients undergoing TKR and TER need rehabilitation to restore limb use, and maximize their functional recovery.

REFERENCES

1. Tomas A, Marcellin-Little DJ, Roe SC, et al. Relationship between mechanical thresholds and limb use in dogs with coxofemoral joint OA-associated pain

and the modulating effects of pain alleviation from total hip replacement on mechanical thresholds. Vet Surg 2014;43:542–8.

2. Lascelles BD, Freire M, Roe SC, et al. Evaluation of functional outcome after BFX total hip replacement using a pressure sensitive walkway. Vet Surg 2010;39:71–7.

3. Brown DC. The canine orthopedic index. Step 1: devising the items. Vet Surg 2014;43:232–40.

4. Valentin S. Cincinnati orthopaedic disability index in canines. Aust J Physiother 2009;55:288.

5. Gingerich DA, Strobel JD. Use of client-specific outcome measures to assess treatment effects in geriatric, arthritic dogs: controlled clinical evaluation of a nutraceutical. Vet Ther 2003;4:376–86.

6. Palmer RH. External fixators and minimally invasive osteosynthesis in small animal veterinary medicine. Vet Clin North Am Small Anim Pract 2012;42:913–34, v–vi.

7. Hawker GA, Badley EM, Borkhoff CM, et al. Which patients are most likely to benefit from total joint arthroplasty? Arthritis Rheum 2013;65:1243–52.

8. Bjorgul K, Novicoff WM, Saleh KJ. Evaluating comorbidities in total hip and knee arthroplasty: available instruments. J Orthop Traumatol 2010;11:203–9.

9. Slaven EJ. Prediction of functional outcome at six months following total hip arthroplasty. Phys Ther 2012;92:1386–94.

10. Peck JN, Liska WD, DeYoung DJ, et al. Clinical application of total hip replacement. In: Peck JN, Marcellin-Little DM, editors. Advances in small animal total joint replacement. Ames (IA): Wiley-Blackwell; 2013. p. 69–107.

11. Marcellin-Little DJ, DeYoung BA, Doyens DH, et al. Canine uncemented porous-coated anatomic total hip arthroplasty: results of a long-term prospective evaluation of 50 consecutive cases. Vet Surg 1999;28:10–20.

12. Dyce J, Wisner ER, Wang Q, et al. Evaluation of risk factors for luxation after total hip replacement in dogs. Vet Surg 2000;29:524–32.

13. Nelson LL, Dyce J, Shott S. Risk factors for ventral luxation in canine total hip replacement. Vet Surg 2007;36:644–53.

14. Malik A, Maheshwari A, Dorr LD. Impingement with total hip replacement. J Bone Joint Surg Am 2007;89:1832–42.

15. Preston CA, Schulz KS, Vasseur PB. Total hip arthroplasty in nine canine hind limb amputees: a retrospective study. Vet Surg 1999;28:341–7.

16. Bergh MS, Gilley RS, Shofer FS, et al. Complications and radiographic findings following cemented total hip replacement: a retrospective evaluation of 97 dogs. Vet Comp Orthop Traumatol 2006;19:172–9.

17. Liska WD. Femur fractures associated with canine total hip replacement. Vet Surg 2004;33:164–72.

18. McCulloch RS, Roe SC, Marcellin-Little DJ, et al. Resistance to subsidence of an uncemented femoral stem after cerclage wiring of a fissure. Vet Surg 2012;41: 163–7.

19. Montgomery RD, Milton JL, Pernell R, et al. Total hip arthroplasty for treatment of canine hip dysplasia. Vet Clin North Am Small Anim Pract 1992;22:703–19.

20. Andrews CM, Liska WD, Roberts DJ. Sciatic neurapraxia as a complication in 1000 consecutive canine total hip replacements. Vet Surg 2008;37:254–62.

21. Liska WD, Doyle ND. Canine total knee replacement: surgical technique and one-year outcome. Vet Surg 2009;38:568–82.

22. Allen MJ, Leone KA, Lamonte K, et al. Cemented total knee replacement in 24 dogs: surgical technique, clinical results, and complications. Vet Surg 2009;38: 555–67.

23. Déjardin LM, Guillou RP, Conzemius M. Clinical application of total elbow replacement in dogs. In: Peck JN, Marcellin-Little DJ, editors. Advances in small animal total joint replacement. Ames (IA): Wiley-Blackwell; 2013. p. 179–98.
24. Jay AR, Krotscheck U, Parsley E, et al. Pharmacokinetics, bioavailability, and hemodynamic effects of trazodone after intravenous and oral administration of a single dose to dogs. Am J Vet Res 2013;74:1450–6.
25. Gruen ME, Roe SC, Griffith E, et al. Use of trazodone to facilitate postsurgical confinement in dogs. J Am Vet Med Assoc 2014;245:296–301.
26. Ewell M, Griffin C, Hull J. The use of focal knee joint cryotherapy to improve functional outcomes after total knee arthroplasty: review artiolo. PM R 2014;6:729–38.
27. Ni SH, Jiang WT, Guo L, et al. Cryotherapy on postoperative rehabilitation of joint arthroplasty. Knee Surg Sports Traumatol Arthrosc 2014. [Epub ahead of print]. http://dx.doi.org/10.1007/s00167-014-3135-x.
28. Büyükyilmaz F, Asti T. The effect of relaxation techniques and back massage on pain and anxiety in Turkish total hip or knee arthroplasty patients. Pain Manag Nurs 2013;14:143–54.
29. Glassner PJ, Slover JD, Bosco JA 3rd, et al. Blood, bugs, and motion—what do we really know in regard to total joint arthroplasty? Bull NYU Hosp Jt Dis 2011;69: 73–80.
30. Turner TM, Urban RM, Sumner DR, et al. Bone ingrowth into the tibial component of a canine total condylar knee replacement prosthesis. J Orthop Res 1989;7: 893–901.
31. Conzemius MG, Aper RL, Corti LB. Short-term outcome after total elbow arthroplasty in dogs with severe, naturally occurring osteoarthritis. Vet Surg 2003;32: 545–52.
32. Van Der Meulen G. Biomechanical considerations in total elbow development. In: Peck JN, Marcellin-Little DJ, editors. Advances in small animal total joint replacement. Ames (IA): Wiley-Blackwell; 2013. p. 164–78.
33. Liska WD, Doyle N, Marcellin-Little DJ, et al. Total hip replacement in three cats: surgical technique, short-term outcome and comparison to femoral head ostectomy. Vet Comp Orthop Traumatol 2009;22:505–10.
34. Woodman JL, Black J, Nunamaker DM. Release of cobalt and nickel from a new total finger joint prosthesis made of vitallium. J Biomed Mater Res 1983;17: 655–68.
35. Sharp B. Feline physiotherapy and rehabilitation: 2. clinical application. J Feline Med Surg 2012;14:633–45.
36. Sharp B. Feline physiotherapy and rehabilitation: 1. principles and potential. J Feline Med Surg 2012;14:622–32.
37. Kramer JF, Speechley M, Bourne R, et al. Comparison of clinic- and home-based rehabilitation programs after total knee arthroplasty. Clin Orthop Relat Res 2003;225–34.

Orthoses and Exoprostheses for Companion Animals

Denis J. Marcellin-Little, DEDV[a],*, Marti G. Drum, DVM, PhD[b],
David Levine, PT, PhD, DPT, CCRP, Cert. DN[c], Susan S. McDonald, EdD, OTR/L[d]

KEYWORDS

- Prosthetic device • Orthosis • Orthotics • Exoprosthesis • Socket prosthesis
- Prosthetic design • Prosthetic fitting • Prosthetic training

KEY POINTS

- Orthoses are external devices that are placed around complete limbs to protect or support them.
- Exoprostheses are likely to be successful when the limb has a functional elbow or stifle joint and a portion of the antebrachium or crus. The longer the stump, the easier it is to fit an exoprosthesis.
- The fabrication and fit of orthotic or prosthetic devices for companion animals must be precise for the device to be stable when worn.
- Axial, angular, and rotational (torsional) stability are key to successful use of an orthosis or exoprosthesis.
- Training companion animals to use an external device is akin to managing limb disuse. It requires patience and attention to details.

Exoprostheses (also named *socket prostheses* or *prosthetics*) are devices that are secured to incomplete limbs to enable locomotion. By comparison, orthoses (also named *orthotics*) are devices externally applied to support or protect an injured body part. Orthoses also can be used to control, guide, protect, limit motion of, or immobilize an extremity, joint, or body segment. Exoprostheses and orthoses are a growing aspect of the physical rehabilitation of companion animals.[1] In veterinary medicine, orthoses may be used to restrict movement in a given direction, such as limiting shoulder abduction with medial shoulder instability, or hip abduction after a ventral hip luxation. They may assist in a movement, such as a carpal or tarsal brace

[a] Department of Clinical Sciences, College of Veterinary Medicine, North Carolina State University, NCSU CVM VHC #2563, 1052 William Moore Drive, Raleigh, NC 27607-4065, USA; [b] Department of Small Animal Clinical Sciences, College of Veterinary Medicine, University of Tennessee, 2407 River Drive, Knoxville TN 37996, USA; [c] Department of Physical Therapy, Dept. #3253, 615 McCallie Avenue, Chattanooga, TN 37403-2598, USA; [d] Department of Occupational Therapy (McDonald), Dept. #3103, 615 McCallie Avenue, Chattanooga, TN 37403-2598, USA
* Corresponding author. NCSU CVM VHC #2563, 1052 William Moore Drive, Raleigh, NC 27607.
E-mail address: djmarcel@ncsu.edu

Vet Clin Small Anim 45 (2015) 167–183
http://dx.doi.org/10.1016/j.cvsm.2014.09.009
0195-5616/15/$ – see front matter © 2015 Elsevier Inc. All rights reserved.
vetsmall.theclinics.com

with nerve injury to the radial or peroneal nerve, respectively. Orthoses also may serve a protective function, such as a tarsal brace after fracture or dislocation, and surgical repair when regional tissues (eg, ligaments, joint capsule, periarticular tendons) are not strong enough to provide the needed support during the healing phase.

ORTHOSES

Orthoses are externally applied devices used to support or protect an injured body part. Orthotics also can be used to control, guide, limit, and/or immobilize an extremity, joint, or body segment. In veterinary medicine, orthoses may be used to restrict movement in a given direction, such as limiting shoulder abduction with medial shoulder instability or after a hip luxation. They may assist in a movement, such as a carpal or tarsal brace with nerve injury to the radial or peroneal nerve, respectively. Orthotics also may serve a protective function, such as a tarsal brace after fracture/dislocation, and surgical repair when the tissues (eg, ligaments) are not strong enough to provide the needed support during the healing phase. Orthoses work by applying forces in specific locations on the body, while preventing tissue damage.

Orthotic devices can be rigid, semirigid, or flexible. Rigid orthoses can be fabricated from custom molds or can be prefabricated in several sizes, such as commercial hock splints. Custom orthoses are made from casts of the patient's limb or are fabricated directly on the patient using a moldable thermoplastic polymer (**Fig. 1**). Heat moldable polymers come in numerous varieties depending on the clinical need, and also can be designed for use with aquatic therapy. Knowledge of the principles of orthotic fabrication is necessary to correctly design the device, as well as a good knowledge of the anatomy and pathology. Flexible orthoses are typically made with breathable neoprene. Nylon straps can be added with hook and loop fasteners (Velcro) to strategically reinforce or limit motion in specific areas (**Fig. 2**), such as limiting carpal hyperextension by reinforcing the palmar aspect of the carpus. Orthoses can be hinged to stabilize or limit the motion of joints (**Fig. 3**). Hinged orthoses are custom made because they need to fit precisely. Orthotic prescription should take into account skin integrity and cleanliness, hair coat, and other concurrent diseases or medications that may potentially affect skin strength and thickness, such as Cushing disease or chronic prednisone treatment. Attention must be given to adequate ventilation and ease of cleaning the appliance, especially for long-term use. Orthoses should also be assessed for their effect on function. For example, a brace may work well in standing but may impede a motion, such as sitting or laying down. When fitting a dog with an orthosis, it is essential to assess the orthosis during functional tasks. Most orthoses have a limited life span and require refurbishment or replacement for long-term use (months to years). In some instances, an orthosis is chosen over surgical correction. However, the owner must be educated about the advantages and disadvantages of each approach. Orthoses should not be considered as a replacement for surgery, as there is no current evidence to support efficacy of orthoses in comparison with conditions traditionally managed by surgery in dogs.

Shoulder Orthoses

The most common shoulder orthoses are used for preventing shoulder abduction either as a primary treatment or to provide postoperative support to dogs with medial shoulder instability secondary to rupture of the medial glenohumeral ligament.[2] Common sources for this type of orthosis include DogLeggs Shoulder Stabilization System (Reston, VA, USA) and Phoenix Design Solutions (Ashburn, VA, USA). The shoulder stabilization orthosis is made from breathable neoprene that can be worn continuously

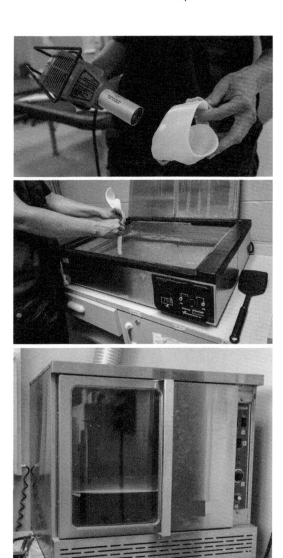

Fig. 1. Thermomoldable polymers are often used to fabricate orthoses and exoprostheses. The polymer can be heated using a hand-held heat gun (*top*), a thermal bath (*center*), or an oven (*bottom*). A polymer sheet is usually heated in an oven or bath, then cut to approximate shape, and contoured on the patient or a positive cast. The shape can be later modified using the heat gun.

during times of activity and rest. As with any orthosis, the device must be examined at least daily for dirt and debris, be kept clean and dry, and the skin under the device checked for abrasion or wounds.

Elbow Orthoses

Elbow luxations have been managed with orthoses, but with limited success, especially in large-breed dogs. Gait retraining is essential in these cases, as abnormal limb position makes reduction difficult. A more common elbow orthosis is for

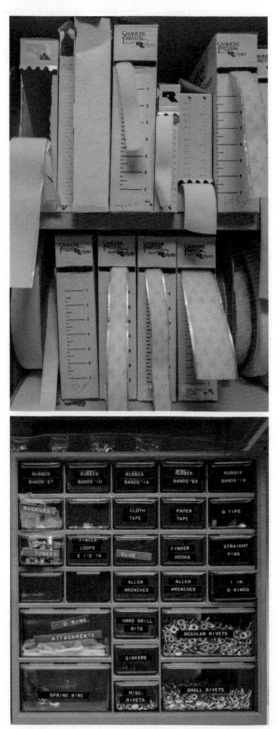

Fig. 2. The supplies needed to fabricate orthoses and exoprostheses include polymers that are shaped to match the limb and closed cell foams that line the polymer (not pictured) that are secured to the body using straps available in multiple materials and widths (*top*). Hinges can be riveted to the shell to form hinged devices. Hinges also are available in several sizes and designs (*bottom*).

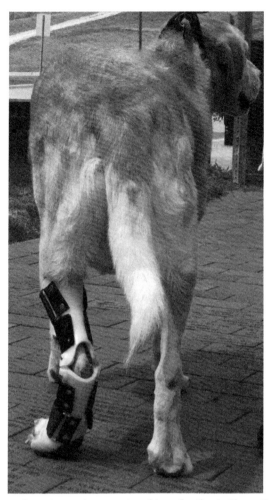

Fig. 3. A Labrador retriever is wearing a custom-hinged orthosis. The orthosis was designed to stabilize an unstable and deformed tarsus that resulted from a chronic joint luxation. The orthosis is open on the caudal aspect of the limb to minimize interference with the calcaneus and common calcanean tendon.

treatment and support of elbow hygromas or elbow decubital ulcers (Elbow Protection; Phoenix Design Solutions, Ashburn, VA, USA or DogLeggs). Elbow protection orthoses resemble shoulder stabilization systems without a band connecting the forelimbs to each other.

Antebrachial and Carpal Orthoses

The most commonly used orthoses in the forelimb are used distal to the elbow. Antebrachial orthotics are uncommon but carpal orthoses are regularly used for mild and moderate carpal hyperextension, for protection after surgery, or for support or management of angular deformities. There is no scientific evidence that carpal orthoses can allow severe carpal hyperextension to heal. Similarly, there is no scientific evidence that carpal orthoses can prevent an increase in bone angulation or torsion that might result from premature closure of one or more radial or ulnar growth plates.

If full carpus immobilization is needed (such as after carpal arthrodesis), a paw shell is an essential feature of the orthosis. An unencumbered paw with rigid support limited to the carpus does not eliminate motion at the carpus. Commercial carpal orthoses can be purchased (Standard Front Leg Splint; OrthoVet, Wilsonville, OR, USA) or custom orthoses can be made by a professional based on a cast of the patient (**Fig. 4**).

Hip Orthoses

Some custom device makers fabricate hip orthoses whose aim is to limit abnormal hip motion or prevent certain hip movement (eg, subluxation). The most common device is the Ehmer sling orthosis (DogLeggs' VEST with Ehmer Sling, Reston, VA, USA). It is different from a typical Ehmer bandage because it is reusable, adjustable, and made of fabric. Other hip orthoses aimed at preventing hip subluxation have limited popularity, and scientific evidence documenting their effectiveness is lacking. They are hindered by the difficulty of application and maintenance of proper position.

Stifle Orthoses

Knee braces are widely used in humans. Some have 1 or 2 rigid hinges, others have no hinge. Knee braces are used to protect the knee after anterior cruciate ligament injuries and medial collateral injuries, to manage the patellofemoral pain syndrome, and to manage pain secondary to osteoarthritis (OA), particularly in patients with unicompartmental (medial compartment) knee pain.[3] Overall, the evidence for the effectiveness of a knee brace in humans is modest.[4] Prophylactic knee braces do not appear to reduce athletic performance or proprioception,[5,6] but their protective value is not known. Hinged braces do not appear to offer advantages after anterior cruciate ligament reconstruction compared with neoprene sleeves.[7] A distraction-rotation knee brace led to functional gait improvement in humans with knee OA.[8] In the long term, distraction knee braces do not appear to decrease the likelihood of total knee replacement in humans with knee OA.[9] A kinematic study evaluating rigid stifle orthoses in dogs demonstrated that cranial tibial translation was not eliminated in a cruciate-deficient canine stifle. However, stifle orthosis have been observed to improve limb use in cranial cruciate ligament ruptures. Some proposed theories to explain this phenomenon are that the orthosis may provide rotational stability, limit flexion enough to discourage a non–weight bearing stance, provide enough partial support during extension to decrease pain, or increase limb awareness. Stifle orthoses alone are not sufficient to improve limb use over the long term. Physical rehabilitation and gait retraining are essential for success in stifle orthotic applications, especially for

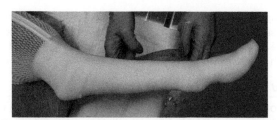

Fig. 4. A cast of the forelimb of a dog with ectrodactyly is being prepared. The dog was sedated. A mesh stockinette was placed around the limb, making sure that the hair was contained within that stockinette. A channel buffer strip was placed along the limb (visible on the left of the image as a yellow strip). The leg was held in a weight-bearing position and semirigid fiberglass was wrapped around the limb. Once the fiberglass has cured, it can be cut using bandage scissors or a carpet knife with a hook blade.

cruciate ligament disease. Neoprene stifle orthoses do not decrease stifle joint insta-bility, but could be useful for improving limb awareness.

Orthoses for patellar luxation are unsuccessful for higher-grade luxations but low-grade patella luxations may respond to orthotic support during targeted exercises. Taping and/or flexible orthotics that are commonly used in low-grade patella luxations of humans are frequently unsuccessful in dogs and cats because skin is highly move-able in dogs and cats. Wounds and skin reaction are a potential complication of taping and flexible patellar luxation orthoses; however, the authors have on rare occasions seen dogs that were managed successfully on a short-term basis.

Hock Orthoses

Hock orthoses are widely used in veterinary medicine. One common use is for the management of calcaneal tendon injuries.[10] Hock orthoses provide support and staged weight bearing after calcaneal tendon repair and conservative management of nonsurgical calcaneal tendon injuries. Hock orthoses are an alternative to (fiber-glass) cast coaptation for calcaneal tendon management when cast sores or regular bandage change become problematic. Hock orthoses also can be used for tarsal instability (see **Fig. 2**), but owners must be educated that the orthotic will likely be needed lifelong. Because of the lack of soft tissue coverage and musculature of the distal crus and tarsus, device sores are common. Clients must be diligent in device maintenance, cleanliness, and skin evaluation to reduce sores, particularly at the prox-imal aspect of the calcaneus (point of the hock).

Distal Limb Orthoses (Distal to Carpus or Tarsus)

Orthoses for the distal limb can be used for metacarpal support, digit immobilization, pad treatments, pad or paw protection, and support for paw deformities.[11,12] A wide number of protective boots (*booties*) are commercially available. Booties are used to protect toes when walking or running on abrasive surfaces (eg, fleece booties worn by sled dogs). The protection of metacarpals/metatarsals and toes in severely paretic or plegic animals is challenging. Most commercially available boots are not designed to have the dorsal aspect dragged or scuffed on the ground. For paretic or plegic ani-mals, a standard boot can be turned around so that the sole of the boot, which is generally reinforced with rubber, Kevlar, or other wear-resistant material, contacts the ground. For animals that are ambulatory, but still scuffing the toe or dorsal paw, Plasti-Dip (Performix, Blaine, MN, USA) or shoe repair kits can be used to create a reinforced toe. However, this application will need to be frequently repeated. Custom boots (TheraPaw, Lebanon, NJ, USA) can be made with a reinforced toe or modifica-tions within the boot for toe or foot issues. Additionally, some prefabricated paw-hock orthoses maintain the foot in a dorsiflexed (extended) position. They are useful in pa-tients with proprioceptive deficits. It is imperative that this specific device approach be used in animals with enough strength to advance the limb or that it only be used with manual assistance during gait retraining/patterning. If used in nonambulatory or weakly ambulatory patients, the weight, decreased sensation, and friction with the ground may actually inhibit movement or worsen ataxia. Ankle orthoses can be used to protect the tarsus in dogs with excessive tarsal extension (**Fig. 5**). Custom ankle-foot orthoses can be used to provide protection over the long term.[12]

Spinal Orthoses

Intervertebral motion can be limited with spinal orthoses. Braces are popular in humans with lumbago, whiplash, and disc herniation, but there is no scientific evi-dence documenting their effectiveness.[13] Spinal braces can be made to limit

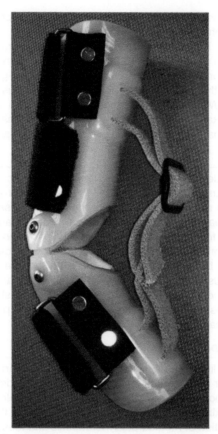

Fig. 5. A custom hinged orthosis has been made to limit tarsal extension in a dog that hyperextended his hock at a walk and trot. The orthosis has an adjustable elastic strap on its cranial side that is used to adjust the tension placed on the pes during extension. It is secured to the limb using 3 straps: 2 around the crus and 1 around the pes.

intervertebral motion in dogs with cervical and thoracic problems, including postoperative brace after surgical stabilization of atlantoaxial subluxation, cervical distraction-fusion, or spinal fracture.

EXOPROSTHESES
Decision Making

Indications

Exoprostheses can be considered as a form of management in companion animals with partial amputations at the proximal third of the antebrachium or mid-crus or distal to these levels. The patients should have a functional shoulder and elbow joints or hip and stifle joints, respectively. Before considering an exoprosthesis, the compatibility of the patient, owner, and medical condition should be evaluated.

The classic indications for exoprostheses include having an incomplete limb because of ectrodactyly (lobster claw deformity), incomplete limb development, traumatic amputation, or surgical amputation. In humans, ectrodactyly may affect 1 or 2 thoracic or pelvic limbs. In dogs and cats, ectrodactyly has been reported only in the thoracic limb, to our knowledge.[14,15] Dogs with ectrodactyly generally lack several digits and metacarpal bones (**Fig. 6**). They often lack carpal stability and have carpal hyperextension. Exoprostheses can be used to protect the abnormal limb and maintain appropriate carpal extension. These socket prostheses are rigid (ie, not hinged). Socket prostheses are also a consideration for patients with partial limbs, regardless of the cause of the loss of limb, provided that none of the contraindications listed in the next section are present. For patients without a carpus and manus (in the forelimb) or without a tarsus and pes (in the pelvic limb), it is difficult to achieve stability without incorporating hinges at the elbow or stifle, respectively. Socket prostheses are particularly indicated when patients have problems in more than one limb, particularly when both forelimbs are abnormal, because locomotion becomes particularly challenging when multiple limbs are abnormal. Patients growing with an incomplete limb generally develop orthopedic problems in the contralateral limb. In the forelimb, these problems may include excessive (rotational) mobility of the shoulder synsarcosis with scapular subluxation, excessive (rotational) mobility of the shoulder joint, and angulation and torsion of the radius. In the pelvic limb, problems resulting from lacking a contralateral limb during growth may include femoral and tibial angulation and torsion, rotational laxity of the stifle, and intertarsal rotational laxity. These problems, subjectively, are more likely to develop in larger and heavier dogs. There is, therefore, an added incentive to fit large growing dogs that have incomplete limbs with socket prostheses as promptly as possible. In cases without elbow joints, a front wheel cart can be used to provide the support and function similar to that of an exoprosthesis.

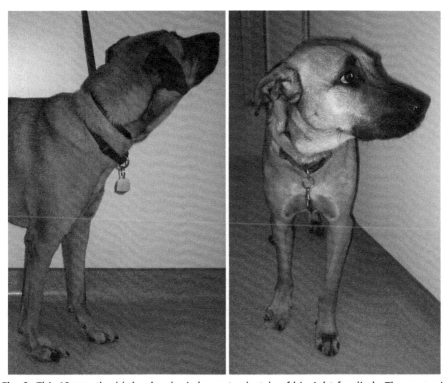

Fig. 6. This 10-month-old shepherd mix has ectrodactyly of his right forelimb. The carpus is slightly unstable, showing signs of hyperextension (*left*) and valgus deviation at a stance (*right*) and walk. The dog was deemed to be a candidate for a custom exoprosthesis.

Contraindications

Contraindications for socket prostheses may be linked to the owner, the patient, or the medical condition. Owner-related contraindications include a potential lack of interest, motivation, supervision, or financial ability to get involved. Patient-related contraindications include being difficult to handle because of an aggressive personality. Having a highly mobile skin in relation to underlying tissues is also a contraindication to socket prostheses. This is particularly true in cats and dogs when patients have a partial amputation below the stifle. Some patients can pull their leg up while their skin is held in place, making it very difficult to secure an exoprosthesis to the residual limb. Excessive skin mobility is unlikely to be an issue in patients with limbs incomplete distal to the carpus or tarsus. Neurologic deficits are a contraindication to wearing an exoprosthesis because neurologically compromised patients usually cannot place their exoprosthesis in a functional position. Compromised joint mobility (eg, contractures) is a contraindication to wearing an exoprosthesis. In patients with partial loss of joint mobility, dynamic hinged braces may be used to stretch a joint. Some of these dynamic hinged braces may potentially be used to improve locomotion. Problems with the residual limbs, including local neoplasia, infection, or stump pain, are relative contraindications to the use of a socket prosthesis. Stump pain may be associated with chronic inflammation, usually as a result of infection, but potentially associated with a nonunion or other problem. A stump also may be painful because of adhesions between the skin and residual bone or because the residual bone is very sharp.

Prosthetic Design and Fabrication

Design

The design of exoprostheses should be adapted to the situation and the technology available to the clinician/prosthetist who will fabricate the device. The decision to incorporate hinges in an exoprosthesis is subjective. Most often, hinged exoprostheses have 2 hinges that are placed over the collateral ligaments of the carpus, elbow, tarsus, or stifle. Hinges may be passive or active. Passive hinges are usually made of nylon (Tamarack Flexure Joint; Tamarack Habilitation Technologies, Blaine, MN, USA). Their size and stiffness vary. Smaller patients need soft passive hinges and larger patients often need stiffer passive hinges. Dynamic hinges may be used when the device needs to provide torque to a joint, usually to stretch it over a long period of time. Dynamic hinges are usually spring-loaded metal hinges. These hinges tend to be very costly. Dynamic hinges may be made using a combination of passive hinges and elastic bands. These are more affordable but they are more bulky and more difficult to fine tune. Most often, passive hinges are incorporated into socket prostheses to address an anticipated lack of stability of the exoprosthesis on the residual limb. Prosthetic stability is a key step in successfully using an exoprosthesis. Stability should be axial (in traction and compression), angular (in medial, lateral, cranio, and caudal bending), and rotational (in internal and external rotation). The addition of passive hinges across the elbow greatly enhances the axial and rotational stability of an exoprosthesis made to replace the distal portion of the antebrachium and manus. Similarly, the addition of passive hinges over the hock greatly increases the stability of exoprostheses made to replace the missing portion of a pes. The longer the stump (also named residual limb or residuum), the easier it is to achieve prosthetic stability. For example, when performing a partial amputation to salvage a limb with a necrotic extremity, it is preferable to spare the calcaneus to counteract rotational forces. The sole of an exoprosthesis should be rounded in craniocaudal and mediolateral directions to optimize locomotion. It should be wear resistant, nonslippery, relatively soft, and lightweight. The fixation of an exoprosthesis should be solid, firm, adjustable, and ergonomic. A rigid or flexible flap or cover may be added to an exoprosthesis to increase its stability. Hook and loop fasteners are used most often for that purpose. The fixation straps should be wide enough to avoid "buckling" of the limb (ie, carpal flexion during weight bearing while the antebrachium and manus are attached to the exoprosthesis). Buckling is prevented by having a fixation strap at the upper and lower parts of the antebrachium and a large fixation strap across the manus.

Casting or scanning the stump

The exoprosthesis is based on a cast of the limb or a 3-dimensional (3D) rendering that may be based on an image captured by a hand-held scanner or a computed tomography (CT) scan. Casting is done either fully awake or under sedation based on clinician or prosthetist preference. Historically (in human prosthetics), casting was done with plaster of Paris because it is safe, comfortable, rapid, and affordable. Plaster of Paris is suboptimal for companion animals because of their hair. The hair and skin are protected by placing a thin stockinette (see **Fig. 4**) or self-adhesive plastic sheet (Glad Press 'N Seal; Glad, Oakland, CA, USA) around the limb. Most clinicians use fiberglass (Scotchcast; 3M, St. Paul, MN, USA) or semi-rigid fiberglass (Scotchcast Soft Cast; 3M, USA) to cast limbs. Semi-rigid fiberglass can be cut by using bandage scissors or a carpet knife with a hook blade. It does not require a cast saw for removal, making the casting process safer for the patient and faster. A casting strip (*channel buffer strip*) may be incorporated into the cast. In small patients, casting strips are not used because they tend to alter the shape of the cast excessively. Fiberglass is cut using a cast saw. Once removed from the limb, the edges of the cast are taped so that the cast retains the shape of the limb while the fiberglass completes the curing process.

As an alternative, a CT scan, handheld 3D scanner, or a smart phone with a 3D capture software application may be used to capture a 3D rendering of the skin surface and a polymer replica of the limb can be made using a 3D printer (**Fig. 7**). Polymer replicas are very accurate[16] and, subjectively, they follow the contours of the skin surface more precisely than casts, particularly in small patients.

Fabrication

The fabrication of socket prostheses is best done by certified orthotists and prosthetists (http://www.abcop.org/). The process often starts with making a positive of the

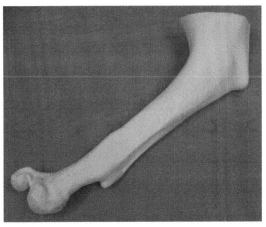

Fig. 7. A replica of the forelimb of a dog with ectrodactyly has been fabricated using fused deposition modeling, a form of 3D printing in which a thin filament of ABS plastic is extruded in thin layers. The leg will be used as a positive to fabricate an exoprosthesis.

stump. The positive is most often made by hand out of plaster of Paris (**Fig. 8**) or can be carved out of a low-density polymer using a computer numerical control machine. Prosthetists typically modify the device on a regular basis, because the stump may change over time or when exoprostheses change due to wear or breakage. Prosthetic fabricators may include 2 versions of a device in the initial fabrication cost to ensure the best fit possible. The positive cast is usually kept for future needs.

Fitting and Training

Initial fit

The initial fit is done by the clinician in a relaxed environment, with the patient awake (ie, not sedated). The patient is placed in lateral recumbency. The hair coat is most often left intact because hair protects the skin from abrasions and ulceration. In some dogs or cats with very long hair, gentle trimming may be necessary to facilitate the placement of a limb in the exoprosthesis. The retaining straps are open and the limb is placed in the exoprosthesis. It may be easier to place the limb in the exoprosthesis from proximal to distal or from distal to proximal, based on shape and tightness. The limb should fit snugly but not tightly. The retaining flap or straps are secured, and the exoprosthesis is manipulated to assess its linear, angular, and rotational stability (**Fig. 9**). There should be no gap or movement of the skin in relation to the device when the exoprosthesis is manipulated. Lack of rotational stability may be addressed by tightening the fixation straps. It the exoprosthesis is too wide, its shape may be modified by changing the shape of the thermoplastic shell or increasing the thickness of foam inserts (**Fig. 10**). It is easier to modify the shape of the portion of the exoprosthesis that surrounds the antebrachium or the crus than the portion of the exoprosthesis that surrounds the manus or pes, because the C-shaped portion that surrounds the antebrachium or crus can be *pinched* to make it fit more tightly. The patient should tolerate the exoprosthesis. Patients that relentlessly lick or chew their exoprostheses most often are experiencing pain or discomfort that is associated with an suboptimal prosthetic fit or with ongoing chronic pain or allodynia.

Initial use

Once the prosthetic fit is satisfactory, patients should stand up to assess the initial limb placement. The initial response to the exoprosthesis varies widely from immediate comfort and weight bearing to a non–weight-bearing lameness with hyperflexion of the hip or shoulder joint. Patients that are weight bearing can move onto the next phase of training aimed at learning to walk. Patients who are non–weight bearing

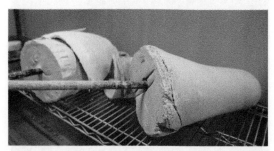

Fig. 8. A positive mold of a stump has been made by filling a cast (negative) of the stump with plaster of Paris. A metal bar is embedded in the cast to secure the positive mold to a work station. Plaster of Paris positive molds are a convenient and cost-effective method to manufacture orthoses and exoprostheses.

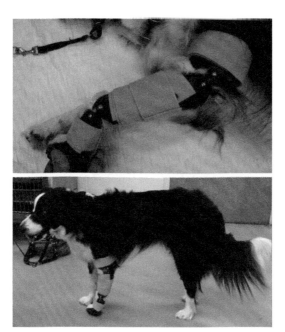

Fig. 9. The initial stability of an exoprosthesis is evaluated by placing the device on the limb with the patient in lateral recumbency (*top*) and by testing the axial (ie, pulling and pushing on the device), angular (ie, bending the device medially, laterally, cranially, and caudally in relation to the limb), and torsional stability (ie, twisting the device internally and externally in relation to the limb) of the device (*top*). If the device is stable, the patient is observed while standing and walking (*bottom*). Some dogs, such as this border collie, use their exoprosthesis immediately. Other dogs need several weeks of training before using their exoprosthesis.

should be treated like patients with limb disuse (ie, dogs that are non–weight bearing after a femoral head ostectomy or after stifle joint surgery) with gentle foot placement in a weight-bearing position and with weight-shifting exercises.[17]

Training
Initial training sessions should last a few minutes and should not be antagonistic so that the patient has a positive experience. It is important to limit the time spent wearing the exoprosthesis if the patient is not bearing weight because the patient can rapidly learn to ambulate without using a limb fitted with an exoprosthesis. Training companion animals to use socket prostheses is akin to managing limb disuse. It relies on habituating patients to tolerate the exoprosthesis at rest and loading it (using it) when standing, when walking slowly (indoors), when walking more rapidly (outdoors), when trotting, when galloping, and then during other activities of daily living (eg, climbing and walking down steps, climbing and walking down stairs, jumping up, jumping down, playing).

ORTHOTIC AND PROSTHETIC MAINTENANCE AND REPAIR
Daily Maintenance

The duration of wear can range widely based on fit and comfort level. Some patients can wear their device all day; others wear it only to go outside for brief walks. The skin integrity and absence of stump or limb pain should be assessed after each removal of

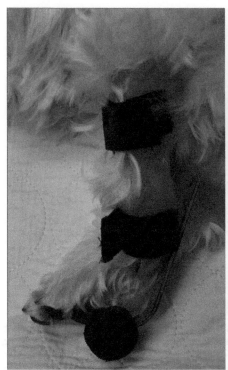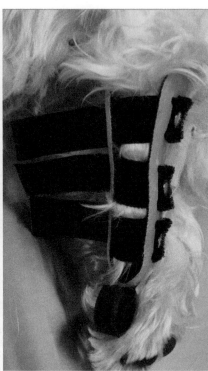

Fig. 10. An exoprosthesis made to replace the missing pes of a West Highland white terrier was initially too loose and too long (*left*). The device was modified by decreasing the width of the thermoplastic shell by 6 mm, by adding a third strap, by creating slots on the medial and lateral aspect of the thermoplastic shell and running the straps through these slots (increasing the holding power of the straps), and by decreasing the length of the pylon connecting the foam sole to the shell. Once modified, the exoprosthesis was stable and was successfully used (*right*).

the device. Hair loss may be a sign of device instability with friction between the limb and the orthosis or exoprosthesis. In patients with short hair, skin redness may precede skin damage in areas of friction or excessive pressure. The device should be modified if skin ulceration occurs. This may be done by slightly altering the shape of the exoprosthesis or by adding foam support in areas surrounding the pressure point, based on the overall fit and tightness of the device. The orthotic or prosthetic should be checked daily and may be cleaned using a mild soap solution (**Fig. 11**). Some manufacturers use a foam that is designed to change color in areas of excessive rubbing, so it must be determined if the device is simply dirty or showing signs of instability or abnormal wear. Hair should be removed from the fasteners. The integrity of the shell, foam, sole, and straps should be assessed.

Repair

One should anticipate wear and tear of an orthosis or exoprosthesis, particularly the sole, when patients are using the device outdoors. The wear of the sole should be used to assess the contact area of the sole and to shape the next sole accordingly. Hinges may wear out and can most often be replaced without needing to construct a new shell. Fasteners that wear out can often be replaced. Foam liners may collapse

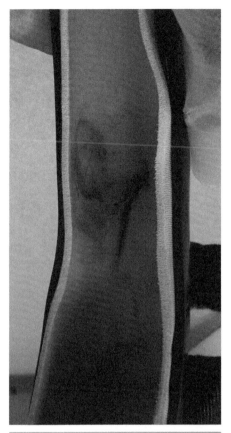

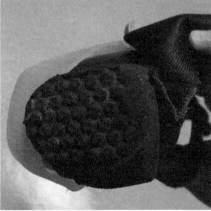

Fig. 11. Orthoses and exoprostheses should be checked daily. A forelimb orthosis is showing a blood stain near the accessory carpal bone (*top*). The skin lesion is most likely the consequence of friction between the skin and orthosis or excessive pressure. Wear on the sole of a prosthetic device indicates that weight bearing occurs on the proximal aspect of the sole (*bottom*).

or crack over time and can often be pulled from the shell and replaced. Dogs and cats can damage their exoprosthesis and it is rarely wise to leave them unattended when they wear their exoprosthesis, even if they have been wearing it successfully for months before.

Altogether, orthoses and exoprostheses require precise design and fabrication. Patients and owners must be trained to use the devices, but they can have a profound beneficial impact on the mobility and the quality of life of companion animals.

REFERENCES

1. Mich PM. The emerging role of veterinary orthotics and prosthetics (V-OP) in small animal rehabilitation and pain management. Top Companion Anim Med 2014;29:10–9.
2. Marcellin-Little DJ, Levine D, Canapp SO Jr. The canine shoulder: selected disorders and their management with physical therapy. Clin Tech Small Anim Pract 2007;22:171–82.
3. Briggs KK, Matheny LM, Steadman JR. Improvement in quality of life with use of an unloader knee brace in active patients with OA: a prospective cohort study. J Knee Surg 2012;25:417–21.
4. Beaudreuil J, Bendaya S, Faucher M, et al. Clinical practice guidelines for rest orthosis, knee sleeves, and unloading knee braces in knee osteoarthritis. Joint Bone Spine 2009;76:629–36.
5. Bottoni G, Herten A, Kofler P, et al. The effect of knee brace and knee sleeve on the proprioception of the knee in young non-professional healthy sportsmen. Knee 2013;20:490–2.
6. Mortaza N, Ebrahimi I, Jamshidi AA, et al. The effects of a prophylactic knee brace and two neoprene knee sleeves on the performance of healthy athletes: a crossover randomized controlled trial. PLoS One 2012;7:e50110.
7. Birmingham TB, Bryant DM, Giffin JR, et al. A randomized controlled trial comparing the effectiveness of functional knee brace and neoprene sleeve use after anterior cruciate ligament reconstruction. Am J Sports Med 2008;36:648–55.
8. Laroche D, Morisset C, Fortunet C, et al. Biomechanical effectiveness of a distraction-rotation knee brace in medial knee osteoarthritis: preliminary results. Knee 2014;21:710–6.
9. Wilson B, Rankin H, Barnes CL. Long-term results of an unloader brace in patients with unicompartmental knee osteoarthritis. Orthopedics 2011;34:e334–7.
10. Case JB, Palmer R, Valdes-Martinez A, et al. Gastrocnemius tendon strain in a dog treated with autologous mesenchymal stem cells and a custom orthosis. Vet Surg 2013;42:355–60.
11. Hardie RJ, Lewallen JT. Use of a custom orthotic boot for management of distal extremity and pad wounds in three dogs. Vet Surg 2013;42:678–82.
12. Levine JM, Fitch RB. Use of an ankle-foot orthosis in a dog with traumatic sciatic neuropathy. J Small Anim Pract 2003;44:236–8.
13. Zarghooni K, Beyer F, Siewe J, et al. The orthotic treatment of acute and chronic disease of the cervical and lumbar spine. Dtsch Arztebl Int 2013;110:737–42.
14. Barrand KR. Ectrodactyly in a West Highland white terrier. J Small Anim Pract 2004;45:315–8.
15. Schneck GW. Two cases of congenital malformation (peromelus ascelus and ectrodactyly) in cats. Vet Med Small Anim Clin 1974;69:1025–6.

16. Fitzwater KL, Marcellin-Little DJ, Harrysson OL, et al. Evaluation of the effect of computed tomography scan protocols and freeform fabrication methods on bone biomodel accuracy. Am J Vet Res 2011;72:1178–85.
17. Marcellin-Little DJ, Freeman J. Rehabilitation after stifle joint surgery. Clinician's Brief 2005;4:39–43. Available at: http://www.cliniciansbrief.com/column/procedures-pro/rehabilitation-after-stifle-joint-surgery.

Feline Rehabilitation

Marti G. Drum, DVM, PhD[a],
Barbara Bockstahler, Dr.med.vet, DVM, PD, CCRP[b],
David Levine, PT, PhD, DPT, CCRP, Cert. DN[c], Denis J. Marcellin-Little, DEDV[d],*

KEYWORDS

- Cat • Physical therapy • Rehabilitation • Therapeutic exercise • Massage
- Ultrasound • Electrical stimulation • Cryotherapy

KEY POINTS

- Cats have orthopedic problems, including osteoarthritis, fractures, and luxations, that are positively impacted by physical rehabilitation.
- Most cats have an independent behavior that requires using a tactful approach to rehabilitation.
- Cats often do well with manual therapy and electrophysical modalities. The sessions may be shorter than canine rehabilitation sessions.
- Cats do best with therapeutic exercises when these exercises are linked to hunting, playing, or feeding.

Physical therapy and rehabilitation is a rapidly growing field in veterinary medicine. In contrast to dogs, feline patients are underrepresented in veterinary physical therapy and rehabilitation. Feline underrepresentation is due to a variety of differences between cats and dogs. Cats appear to have fewer developmental orthopedic diseases and orthopedic injuries as a whole. Also, less is known about orthopedic problems in cats compared with dogs. For example, osteoarthritis (OA) is a well-known problem in dogs but it is only an emerging problem in cats[1]; this is especially problematic because it was proved that most cats (>90% in the age range from 6 months to 20 years, with a high correlation with age) have at least one joint with radiologic signs of degenerative joint disease.[2] One major problem in the detection of OA-related disorders in cats is a mismatch between radiographic prevalence of OA and clinical signs.[1,3] Such a mismatch does not appear to be present in dogs. Cats suffering from chronic pain react with changes of their behavior/lifestyle rather than with lameness like dogs. Cats may also be underrepresented as euthanasia may be elected more frequently in comparison with dogs with similar conditions, due to financial

[a] Department of Small Animal Clinical Sciences, College of Veterinary Medicine, University of Tennessee, 2407 River Drive, Knoxville TN 37996, USA; [b] Department für Kleintiere und Pferde, Veterinärmedizinische Universität, Veterinärplatz 1, 1210 Wien, Austria; [c] Department of Physical Therapy, University of Tennessee at Chattanooga, Dept. #3253, 615 McCallie Avenue, Chattanooga, TN 37403-2598, USA; [d] Department of Clinical Sciences, College of Veterinary Medicine, North Carolina State University, NCSU CVM VHC #2563, 1052 William Moore Drive, Raleigh, NC 27607-4065, USA
* Corresponding author. NCSU CVM VHC #2563, 1052 William Moore Drive, Raleigh, NC 27607
E-mail address: djmarcel@ncsu.edu

Vet Clin Small Anim 45 (2015) 185–201
http://dx.doi.org/10.1016/j.cvsm.2014.09.010
vetsmall.theclinics.com
0195-5616/15/$ – see front matter © 2015 Elsevier Inc. All rights reserved.

reasons, perceived poor outcomes, or poor quality of life even with intervention. Another (false) belief is that cats are not treatable with most methods of physical therapy because of their independent behavior and their potentially low tolerance to handling. However, even if the species-related behavior of cats makes it somewhat trickier to handle the patient, cats have some unique characteristics that can be leveraged in the development of a rehabilitation program and most treatment modalities can be used, once adapted to the special needs of the cats.

Because cats can be impatient, quickly bored, and not as accustomed to restraint or handling as dogs, they are mostly less tolerant than dogs, and therefore, it is more difficult to perform exercises with them. As a result, the time of the session should be as short as possible and offer a variety of different activities that should be adapted to the cat's special behavior. On the other hand, the behavioral characteristics of cats, such as playing and hunting, can be used to design active exercise. It is a delicate balance to anticipate the threshold of what the feline patient may or may not tolerate. If a particular exercise is successful, it is continued as long as possible (as tolerated). The endpoint may be far before fatigue and/or pain dictates the exercise or session should end. The treatments must be chosen with respect to the acceptance and attitude of the cat. Some cats enjoy electrotherapy or ultrasound treatment; some do not. Besides the need to be alert for injuries because of claws or bites if the animal's tolerance threshold has been exceeded, the therapist should be able to choose the most applicable therapy that offers the best medical effect with the best acceptance of the cat. As an example, if a cat does not accept electrical therapy for pain control, perhaps therapeutic laser therapy (**Fig. 1**) is

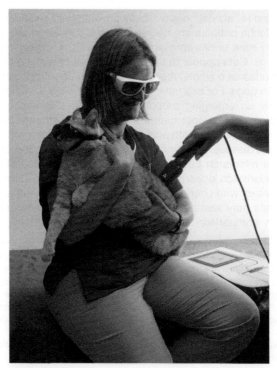

Fig. 1. Therapeutic laser is applied to the painful area of the spine. Certified laser safety glasses must be worn to protect the retina. Clipping of hair in the area is also recommended for maximal effectiveness.

tolerated. In dogs, hydrotherapy is extremely popular for exercise, and almost every dog can be accustomed to the underwater treadmill. Hydrotherapy can be considerably difficult to use in particular cats, but some cats readily accept underwater treadmill exercise.

There are several obvious differences in the pathophysiology of disorders of cats and dogs: as an easy example, cranial cruciate disease in dogs is known as a degenerative disease, whereas in cats it is mostly traumatic and therefore often connected with other ligament, tendon, and surrounding soft tissue damages. Therefore, the therapist must have in-depth knowledge about feline anatomy, physiology of tissues and their healing processes, and the pathophysiology and treatment of the underlying disease to start the different rehabilitative techniques on time, based on tissue strength. Initial baseline evaluations are equally important in cats, and routine orthopedic and neurologic examinations should be part of the initial rehabilitation evaluation. Goniometric indices for cats have been described (**Table 1**).[4] Thigh girth measurement has been described in dogs, and the same technique is currently used in cats, although measurement variability has not been evaluated. An overview of common physical therapy interventions applicable in cats is presented in this article (**Table 2**).

MASSAGE
Principles

Massage has been proven as an effective treatment modality in several conditions, such as low back pain in humans.[5] Massage is often recommended for rehabilitation of small animals.[6] Pain and resulting disuse of limbs can result in considerable muscle tension. As a reaction to the pain, muscles develop an increased tension, which results in reduced local blood flow in the affected region. Subsequently, the oxygen supply to the affected muscles and the removal of metabolic waste products from the muscles

Table 1
Range of motion (degrees) of various joints measured by goniometry in 20 healthy, nonsedated cats

Joint	Position	Mean	SD	95% CI of the Mean	Median
Carpus	Flexion	22	2	22–23	22
	Extension	198	6	196–199	198
	Valgus	10	2	9–10	10
	Varus	7	2	6–7	7
Elbow	Flexion	22	2	22–23	22
	Extension	163	4	162–164	162
Shoulder	Flexion	32	3	31–32	32
	Extension	163	6	162–165	164
Tarsus	Flexion	21	1	21–22	22
	Extension	167	4	166–168	167
	Valgus	7	2	7–8	7
	Varus	10	3	10–11	10
Stifle	Flexion	24	2	24–25	24
	Extension	164	4	163–165	166
Hip	Flexion	33	3	32–33	32
	Extension	164	4	163–165	164

Abbreviations: CI, confidence interval; SD, standard deviation.
From Jaeger GH, Marcellin-Little DJ, Depuy V, et al. Validity of goniometric joint measurements in cats. Am J Vet Res 2007;68:824; with permission.

Table 2
Summary of rehabilitative therapies in cats, including unique considerations and tolerance level in most cats undergoing rehabilitation

Modality	Cats	Special Considerations for Cats
Massage	Mostly well tolerated	Be careful and use only techniques the cat enjoys. Minimal restraint techniques are best for low stress sessions.
Hot packs/infrared lamps	Well tolerated	Infrared lamps allow for minimal or no restraint. Hot packs can be challenging for some cats that do not like to be held or restrained.
Therapeutic ultrasound	Well tolerated	Consider the small amount of soft tissue and use lower intensities and smaller ThUS heads.
Cold	Sometimes	Cold pack application can be sometimes difficult because cats often refuse to remain still for long periods of time. Cryomassage may be preferred if affected area is small.
Electrical stimulation	Often tolerated	Use lower intensity as in dogs. Use electrodes of a size suitable for cats. If necessary, shorten the treatment time.
Therapeutic exercises	Often tolerated	Use the special behavior of cats to introduce exercises like playing and hunting.

Adapted from Levine D, Bockstahler B. Physical therapy and rehabilitation. In: Schmeltzer L, Norsworthy GD, editors. Nursing the feline patient. Ames (IA): Wiley-Blackwell; 2012. p. 138–42; with permission.

are reduced; this leads to a vicious circle of pain, muscle tension, impaired blood flow, and more pain. To break this vicious circle of pain and muscle tension, massage offers many beneficial therapeutic effects, such as the increase of blood flow, increased oxygen supply, and the release of endogenous endorphins. Patients with nerve and muscle disorders can also benefit from massage therapy. Various techniques can be used to increase or decrease muscle tone and to improve conscious awareness of the body.

Indications

Indications include the improvement of muscle spasms secondary to musculoskeletal disorders, physical overexertion, and gait anomalies to increase the blood flow, increase the elasticity of tendons and ligaments, improve the joint and muscle function, and prevent tissue adhesions after surgery. Massage should not be used in the case of tumors, infections, cardiac decompression, fever, or bleeding disorders.

Techniques

Many different massage techniques are described in the literature. The most common or classic "Swedish" techniques are discussed here.[6]

Effleurage

Effleurage, or stroking, is a superficial technique used to increase blood flow and make the animal comfortable with the treatment. The open hands are placed flat on the muscles, starting from the neck and stroking the muscles gently and not too rapidly, proceeding from the neck, down the back, and to the croup and legs. Stroking is used in recumbency (sternal or lateral) to promote relaxation, but can also be applied with the animal standing. This technique is excellent to relax the cat. Stroking should always be performed as a warm-up for the massage session. Stroking also serves to relax the patient between deep tissue manipulation and at the end of a massage session.

Petrissage
Petrissage is a kneading type of massage and is very effective in increasing blood supply, mobilizing tissues, and lengthening fibrous tissues. Petrissage increases the extensibility and strength of connective tissues. Several different types of kneading motions are used. For example, wringing, skin rolling, and pick-up-and-squeeze are all potrissage techniques. Especially when manipulating deeper tissues, kneading can induce pain. Therefore, the pressure must always increase gradually while carefully monitoring the patient's response. It should not be used until the patient is relaxed and the tissues have been warmed, either by touch or by superficial heat. Always loosen the tissues by stroking or shaking between each round of petrissage.

Tapotement
Tapotement, or rhythmic percussion, is usually performed with the edge of the hand, a cupped hand, or the fingertips. Types of tapotement are, for example, tapping (only fingertips are used) or hacking with the edge of the hand. It increases the blood flow, mobilizes muscles and fascia, and helps to facilitate flushing toxins from tissue. In cats, this technique can be sometimes unpleasant and should therefore be used carefully.

Special Considerations in Cats

In general, the therapist should respect the character of cats, should not stress the cat through handling, and should therefore not restrain the cat more than what is absolutely necessary. Most cats will relax and enjoy the treatment if they have enough time to acclimate.

USE OF HEAT
Principles

Heat can be applied to increase the release of mediators such as histamine, bradykinin, and prostaglandins, resulting in the dilation of blood vessels and an increase in the metabolic rate of tissues. It further increases the extensibility of fibrous tissues, such as ligaments, tendons, and scar tissue.

Indications

Heat therapy is mainly used to treat chronic diseases and to warm up the body before active and passive exercise or massage. It is useful in patients with OA, back pain due to spondylarthrosis, lumbosacral disease (or other lumbar spine conditions), or muscle spasms, and to prepare tissues such as muscles and tendons for exercise. Contraindications are acute inflammation, tumors, open wounds, and severe cardiac insufficiency. Caution should be used in areas with decreased or absent sensation.

Techniques

To heat tissues up to a depth of 2 cm, commercially available hot packs can be used. The hot pack should be heated only to the point that it is comfortable to the therapist's touch and is not too hot. To prevent skin burns, hot packs should be wrapped in a towel or cloth, not placed directly on the skin. They are applied to the affected body part for 15 to 20 minutes, 1 to 3 times daily. Infrared heat lamps are used to warm large areas of the body. Position any commercially available infrared heat lamp 30 to 40 cm from the affected area. Because tissue temperature rapidly decreases after removal of superficial heat, stretching and range of motion (ROM) exercises should be performed during or immediately after heating.[6]

Special Considerations in Cats

Most cats like the application of heat, especially the use of infrared lamps, whereas the use of hot packs is sometimes difficult because cats often object to lying quietly with a hot pack on a joint or the back. Many sociable cats prefer to lie in a lap or be held while hot packs are applied. A swaddling technique with a towel is useful as a low-stress restraint technique for hot-pack application.

THERAPEUTIC ULTRASOUND
Principles

As described above, hot packs and infrared lamps are useful to heat tissues up to maximum depth of 2 cm. For deep tissue heating in veterinary physical therapy, therapeutic ultrasound (ThUS) is the commonly used modality to improve the extensibility of connective tissues, to decrease pain and muscle spasms, and to promote tissue healing and improve the quality of scar tissue. The biological effects of ultrasound differ depending on the used mode: using a continuous mode, the thermal effects are maximized and it is therefore primarily used for tissue heating before stretching. If pulsed ThUS mode is used, the thermal effects are decreased but other effects occur based on the phase of tissue repair, including the acceleration of the inflammatory process, increased fibroblast proliferation, and increasing tensile strength of healing tissues.

Indications

Typical indications for ThUS are the increasing of the tissue temperature before stretching, the treatment of calcifying tendinitis, and the acceleration of the wound-healing process. It should not be used over the spinal cord after laminectomy, over the epiphyseal area of immature physis, over the heart or in animals with peacemakers, in areas at risk for embolism, and over tumors or infections.

Techniques

Principally 2 modes of ultrasound are available: continuous modes (100%) and pulsed modes (typically 20% duty cycle). The mode is chosen based on the desired effects: thermal effects are most pronounced with continuous mode, whereas tissue-healing effects are achieved when a pulsed mode is used. For deeper tissues up to a depth of 2 to 5 cm, 1 MHz ThUS is used; for more superficial tissues (0–3 cm of depth), 3.3 MHz ThUS is used.[7] The intensity for ultrasound ranges between 0.5 W/cm^2 (small amount of soft tissue) and 1.5 W/cm^2 (large amount of soft tissue). The size of the area to be treated and of the sound head dictates the treatment time. In general, 4 minutes of treatment are necessary for each sound head that fits into the treatment area (eg, ThUS head size of 5 cm^2, treatment area of 10 cm^2: treatment time of 8 minutes). The hair must be clipped for effective transmission and to avoid skin burns.[8]

Special Considerations in Cats

Cats principally tolerate ThUS very well, but a small ThUS head must be used to ensure the plane positioning of the sound head over the treatment area. Also important to consider is that cats have less soft tissue than dogs, and lower intensities should be used in cats compared with dogs.

USE OF COLD
Principles

The application of cold (or cryotherapy) causes vasoconstriction and therefore reduces bleeding in the area after injury or surgery. Cold also decreases the metabolism of cells, decreases nerve conduction velocity, and helps to alleviate pain. It decreases the impulse conduction velocity and stimulates cold receptors, thereby activating the gate control system via neural mechanisms.[9]

Indications

Cold is used to decrease swelling, pain, and the overall inflammatory process after surgery and exercise and to reduce swelling and pain in acute stages of OA, for example. Cold should not be used in patients with paraesthesia or circulatory disorders.[9]

Techniques

Commercially available cold packs or ice packs can be used to cool tissues. They are typically wrapped in a thin towel and placed directly on the affected body part for about 15 to 20 minutes 1 to 3 times daily.

Special Considerations in Cats

As described for heat, it might be sometimes difficult to place the cold pack on the target area because cats sometimes refuse to lie quietly for more than a few minutes. Nevertheless, the therapist should try to use cold, especially in the early phase after surgery.

ELECTROTHERAPY
Principles

Orthopedic and neurologic diseases causing acute and chronic pain, or muscle atrophy, are often treated using electrical stimulation (ES). ES is a useful therapeutic modality and is often possible in cats. In fact, many cats enjoy this modality. Nevertheless, cats must be introduced carefully to ES in order for them to become familiar with ES. Principally, ES can be used for muscle strengthening and pain control. Neuromuscular electrical stimulation is a form of ES whereby current is used to stimulate a motor nerve and cause the contraction of a muscle or muscle group. To stimulate a denervated muscle (eg, in patients with spinal cord injuries), the muscle fibers must be excited directly and the ES is then called electrical muscle stimulation. For pain control, analgesia occurs because of several mechanisms such as the gate control theory and the release of endogenous endorphins. The most commonly used type of ES for pain control is transcutaneous electrical nerve stimulation.[9] The biological effects of ES depend on the parameters used, including frequency and intensity, and the type of motor responses (single twitches using low frequencies, tetanic contractions with higher frequencies, and myokymia), hyperemia due to muscle work and release of vasodilators and analgesia due to activation of gate control system, reduction of muscle tone, stimulation of blood flow, and release of endogenous endorphins.[10]

Indications

Many conditions affecting cats are amenable to ES. Cats suffering from OA or spondylarthrosis or recovering from orthopedic or neurosurgery can benefit from ES.

Precautions/contraindications include anesthetized areas of skin, acute inflammation, infection, and tumors.

Techniques

Different electrodes are available for use in humans and animals. Most have a rubberized or gel surface but needle electrodes are also available. With the exception of needle electrodes, the hair coat should be clipped before treatment to lower impedance and decrease the amount of current needed for effect. A suitable contact medium, such as ultrasound gel, may be applied to ensure a complete contact between skin and electrodes. To elicit muscle contractions, the electrodes are placed near the motor point and the muscle-tendon junction, respectively. For pain treatment, the electrodes can be placed directly on the painful area, segmentally via the spinal nerve root innervating the target tissue or over acupuncture/trigger points.

Special Considerations in Cats

The procedure is basically the same as described for dogs, with the several differences. The treatment should always be started with a form of current perceived as pleasant and the used intensity is generally lower than in dogs. There is a need to use electrodes of a smaller size as in most small dogs and it may be necessary to shorten treatment time.[6]

THERAPEUTIC EXERCISES FOR CATS
Principles

Therapeutic exercises (TE) are one of the most important aspects of the rehabilitation process. To properly design an exercise program, exercises should be selected based on the stage of tissue repair to avoid any risk to worsen the symptoms. It is therefore mandatory that the therapist understands the underlying pathologic condition, the expected recovery progress, and the biomechanics of cats.

Indications

TE are performed to improve the passive and active ROM of joints, to increase muscle mass and strength, to improve conditioning and endurance, to increases limb use, to enhance proprioceptive re-education, to improve quality of gait movements, to increase mobility, and to improve daily function. TE are contraindicated if the desired movement could worsen the state of the disorders (eg, high impact exercises in acute cases of OA or directly after fracture stabilization).

Techniques

A unique challenge of therapeutic exercise prescription in cats is to select appropriate patients.[6] Even fractious patients can be amenable to therapy with low-stress handling techniques. A greater challenge is the fearful cat because they frequently will curl into a ball and refuse to move or cooperate in any way, choosing passive resistance instead. In some instances, the lure of a crate or cat carrier can be appropriate motivation to encourage movement of all cats. Pheromone spray is another useful tool to encourage cooperation for therapeutic exercise. TE can be divided into passive exercises, proprioceptive training exercises, and active exercises.[6]

Passive exercises are performed without an active muscle contraction of the patient and help to maintain or improve the ROM of joints, improve flexibility of muscles, tendons, and ligaments, and help enhance awareness of neuromuscular structure and function.[11] Passive ROM exercises are very useful in cats and kittens undergoing any joint surgery, especially stifle surgery, elbow fractures, and fractures of the distal femoral physis. For passive ROM exercises, a joint is moved without an active muscle contraction of the patient within the comfortable ROM and is therefore performed to maintain the flexibility of joints, not to increase the flexibility, muscle strength, or endurance. Usually, all joints in the affected limb are treated, starting distally, and 10 to 30 repetitions can be performed 2 to 3 times daily. More natural gait movement may be instituted by putting all of the joints of a limb through an ROM simultaneously, for example, performing *bicycling exercises.* This exercise is performed to train the passive ROM of the joints and gait patterns and can be performed in lateral recumbency or in a standing position (in which case the animal should be assisted to prevent falling). The tarsal or carpal region is grasped gently and the limb is moved smoothly in circular caudal to dorsal to cranial movements. Passive ROM exercises are performed to maintain joint mobility. To increase the flexibility of joints and periarticular tissues (such as the joint capsule, tendons, and muscles), *stretching* exercises are performed. The joint is flexed until a restriction is detected and the muscles and connective tissues are stretched (**Fig. 2**). The stretch is held for 20 to 30 seconds. The same procedure is repeated in extension direction. Exercises are repeated for 2 to 5 times, 1 to 3 times daily. As cats are quickly bored and refuse sometimes to hold a certain limb position over a longer period of time and often do not like manual manipulation of the limbs, it may be more effective and safer for the therapist to use the cat's body weight than performing passive stretching exercises (**Fig. 3**).

If the cat is able to bear some of its body weight, *assisted exercises* can be introduced. For example, *assisted standing* is a valuable exercise after orthopedic and neurologic surgery. Assisted standing trains neuromuscular function and proprioception while simultaneously improving strength and endurance of the cat in a standing position. To support the cat, the therapist's hands are often the most useful, but body slings, harnesses, or support rolls (Physio Roll, pillow, or rolled towel) can be used (**Fig. 4**). Care should take that the limbs are placed squarely underneath the body. Cat claws can puncture Physio Rolls and balls and the material needs to be covered with a towel or padding if the claws are likely to contact it directly. The cat should bear as much weight as possible for several seconds. As soon the cat shows signs of weakness, it is lifted back into a standing position. As the cat becomes stronger, the therapist provides less support. Repeat for 5 to 15 repetitions, 1 to 3 times daily. *Weight-shifting exercises* are an excellent exercise to improve balance,

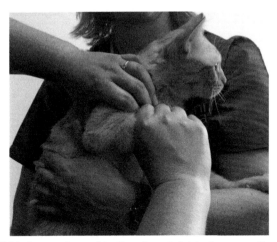

Fig. 2. Passive ROM being performed to the elbow joint to improve elbow flexion motion.

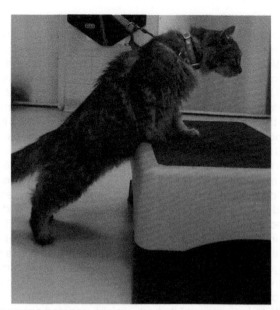

Fig. 3. A cat with limited hip extension performing a functional stretch using their body weight and a tracking game. A toy is held in front of the cat and the harness is used to control their position.

proprioception, and the use of a limb. They can be introduced as soon the cat is able to stand safely. The therapist tries to disturb the balance by gently pushing the animal on the shoulder or the pelvis momentarily, causing a loss of stability for the cat. Adding an unstable surface such as a balance board (**Fig. 5**), balance pad, foam bed, or balance disk may be needed for some difficult cases or as a progression of the exercise from level ground. This exercise should be repeated for 5 to 15 repetitions, 1 to 3 times daily. *Wheelbarrowing exercises* are used to improve the use of the forelimbs and to strengthen or stretch the forelimb muscles. The rear legs are lifted off the ground and the cat is moved forward. *Dancing* (**Fig. 6**) can be performed to improve use and muscle strength or ROM of the hind legs. The forelimbs are lifted off and the cat is encouraged to move several steps forward and/or backward.

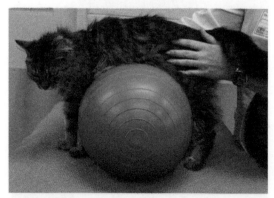

Fig. 4. Supported (assisted) standing over a Physio Roll to build endurance and muscle strength and to enhance balance and proprioception.

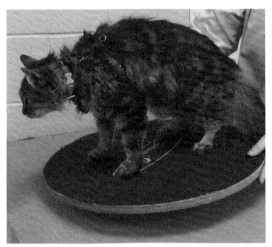

Fig. 5. Balance board/platform being used to challenge balance, promote limb use, and also provide strengthening.

Cats may be difficult to motivate, but some of their playing and hunting behaviors can be used to design *active exercises*. For example, many cats will readily chase a *laser light beam* (**Fig. 7**) or feather on a string around a room and moving the light along the wall can motivate the cat to stretch the legs to reach the light. Laser lights can also be useful for land treadmill training in appropriately motivated cats. Good footing, such

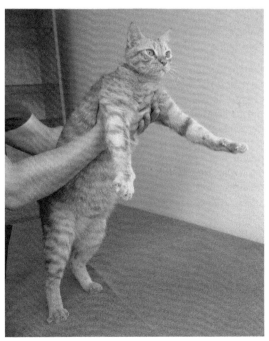

Fig. 6. Dancing exercises used to promote rear limb use. This exercise can be performed forward or backward depending on the muscles or joints affected.

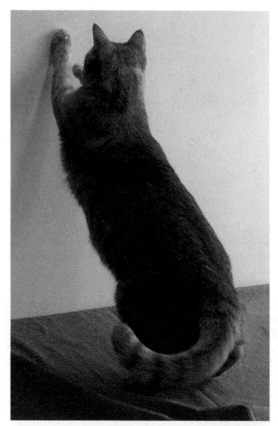

Fig. 7. Laser beam light being used in rehabilitation to increase hip extension ROM.

as carpeting, is essential. Caution should be used to move the light at a speed appropriate for that animal's stage of recovery. *Playing with a toy mouse*, string, or any other toy the cat likes is useful to encourage ROM activities of the limbs. For example, to train the ROM of the forelimbs, the toy may be dangled at a height so that the cat sits on its hind limbs while using the forelimbs to "catch" the toy. To encourage use of the forelimbs and hind limbs, the toy may be dragged along the ground at a distance so that the cat chases and "pounces" on the toy. Another possibility is crawling through tunnels, which encourages the flexion of all limb joints. Dragging a toy around chair legs forces the side bending of the spine.

Aquatic therapy

Cats tolerate aquatic therapy surprisingly well. It can be a very useful tool during the rehabilitation of many cats. Patient selection is the most important criterion. Cats may struggle with aquatic-based therapy, and it could potentially lead to further injury. However, these cats are also likely to be difficult rehabilitation patients overall. Specific breeds, such as Bengal cats, are naturally attracted to water and can be excellent patients for aquatic therapy. In addition, the popularity of nondomesticated felines as pets (Servals and Savannah cats) can provide particular challenges, and these cats are often easier to handle in aquatic therapy because of their natural inclination toward water. Specifically, with an underwater treadmill, it is often not the water that is problematic but the moving belt of the treadmill that creates hesitation to walk. In such a case, it may be useful for the therapist to be in the underwater treadmill for the initial sessions and begin with walking back and forth in the treadmill chamber without turning on the belt. A life jacket is considered required for the first session until the cat's reaction can be determined. Subsequent sessions can use a small harness instead because some cats will object to the bulkiness of life jackets (**Fig. 8**). As mentioned previously, short sessions are essential. However, this must be balanced with the tendency of cats to grow progressively bored or resistant of a particular exercise. Motivation is essential for training, and using an enticing treat such as salmon paste (Kong Stuff'N Easy Treat, Kong, Golden, CO, USA) or shredded chicken is recommended during initial training during breaks for positive reinforcement.

Underwater treadmill training

Often, even food-motivated cats will not eat when stressed, so stopping the treadmill belt can be used as a positive reinforcement along with verbal praise. Initially, when beginning to move the belt, support and encourage the patient until it takes only 1 or 2 steps forward voluntarily; then stop the belt immediately. This process may only take 5 or 10 seconds, but it should be repeated 2 or 3 times until challenging the cat with a longer duration of up to 1 minute. Many cats will only tolerate only 1- or 2-minute intervals for several assisted sessions regardless of fitness or mobility levels. Also, begin with a very slow speed (often the slowest speed possible), usually no more than 0.23 m/s (0.5 mph). Vary the water level initially to find the level where the cat will walk forward voluntarily; then increase slowly to the desired level. Many cats will resist and float their hind limbs or try climbing out of the treadmill with higher water levels. As the patient improves, lowering the water level will increase resistance, which can be advantageous for increasing ROM or aerobic activity.

Swimming

It is recommended to start all cats in the underwater treadmill first for water acclimation, as swimming is more challenging and less tolerable to many cats. Again, a life jacket is required for initial introduction to the swimming pool. It also provides a handle to guide and control the patient (**Fig. 9**). It is favorable to allow the patient to swim to a point and return to a resting spot compared with swimming in place. Eventually, manual resistance to slow the cat and prolong duration of swimming can be worked up to. Begin with very short, 2- to 5-minute sessions, when training. Frequently,

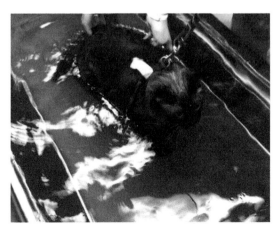

Fig. 8. A cat in an underwater treadmill with life vest on for buoyancy and for control by the handler.

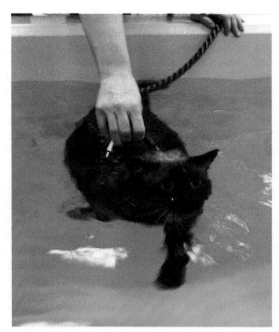

Fig. 9. A cat swimming in a pool. The cat swims to the length of its leash and then returns to the start.

cats will tolerate the first 1 or 2 sessions, but become increasingly dismayed with swimming.

SPECIFIC INJURIES/SURGERIES
Traumatic Stifle Luxation

Traumatic stifle luxation was formerly referred to as a *deranged stifle*. Traumatic stifle luxation is more common in cats than dogs and is the result of a major trauma, such as a motor vehicle accident, a dog attack, the affected hind limb being caught in a fan belt, fence, or other event where the cat is trapped by the hind limb.[12] Several methods have been reported to stabilize luxated stifles, including rigid immobilization with transarticular pinning or external fixator for 6 weeks or more to allow stifle fibrosis and stability.[12,13] Although cats can be functional with repair following traumatic stifle luxation, rehabilitation following removal of a transarticular pin or external fixator is very important and can be very rewarding. TE initially focus on flexion-based activities combined with modalities to improve passive ROM, which can begin immediately following implant removal. Progression to active extension and flexion-based activities once strength and ROM begins to improve may be started as soon as tolerated, possibly within the first week of implant removal. Cavaletti rails, tunnels, climbing stairs, inclines or kitty condos, balance board, and aquatic therapy are effective activities to achieve functional mobility. Hinged linear external skeletal fixators have also been used to stabilize traumatic stifle luxations.[14] Hinged linear external fixators preserve more joint motion during postoperative recovery and therefore facilitate the rehabilitation process after frame removal.

Femoral Fractures

Cats of any age are at risk of contracture of the quadriceps femoris muscle following distal femur fractures.[15] Prevention is key, because loss of stifle flexion is frequently irreversible or only treatable with adhesion release/revision and aggressive physical therapy. Cast immobilization has been shown to be unsuccessful in managing feline femur fractures, and quadriceps contracture is associated with cast immobilization for treatment of femur fracture.[15] Quadriceps contracture can occur with internal fixation as well; 4 of 28 cats with a femoral fracture had a quadriceps contracture in one retrospective study.[16] It is far easier to educate the client regarding the early signs of quadriceps contracture, diligently assess stifle flexion in the first 2 weeks after surgery, and advocate early passive ROM and weight-bearing activities in the immediate postoperative period (beginning in the first 24 hours after surgery). Severe soft tissue trauma (either from the original traumatic accident or surgically induced) increases the risk of quadriceps contracture, and in those cases hospitalization is recommended for 3 to 7 days after surgery for aggressive rehabilitation, until active flexion of the stifle joint is present (see the article by Marcellin-Little and Levine in this issue).

Femoral Head and Neck Excision

As in dogs, femoral head and neck excision is a common treatment in cats for disorders of the hip, such as avascular necrosis of the femoral head, femoral capital physeal fractures, hip dislocation, and OA. Early weight-bearing is essential and limited hip extension will have a direct effect on weight-bearing due to pain and mechanical limitations. Many cats are in too much pain to tolerate aggressive passive ROM in the postoperative period, so often active ROM in combination with very gentle passive ROM is used during recovery. Although sit-to-stand exercises can be difficult with cats, this exercise is often successful if done with meal feedings. The cat must "earn" their meals as many cats will sit or lie down to eat without command. The meal is then moved a few feet so that the cat must stand up and walk to the food. This exercise is often more easily accomplished with canned food. If using dry food, only place 2 or 3 pieces of kibble in the dish at a time. Other activities to improve hind-end strength are applicable as well, such as stretching into hip extension using a ball or roll (**Fig. 10**).

Articular Fractures

Regardless of species, articular fractures are particularly problematic because of excessive scar tissue formation, joint capsule fibrosis, and intra-articular

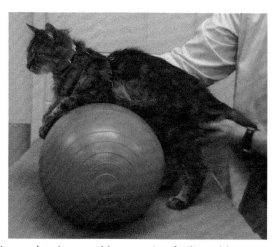

Fig. 10. An exercise used to increase hip extension facilitated by using a ball or roll. The higher the ball or roll, the more hip extension required.

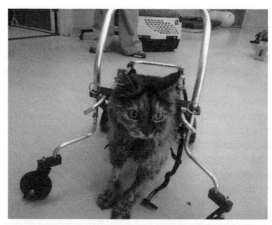

Fig. 11. A tetraparetic cat is walking assisted by a quad cart. The cart has front wheels that are spaced apart to increase stability. The front wheels swivel to facilitate turning.

inflammation. Early intervention is necessary to reduce the debilitating sequelae common to articular fractures. Exercise should be proportional to the severity of fracture and loss of ROM. Thus, it is essential that proper follow-up and client education to identify loss of ROM, increasing lameness, and evaluation of pain are critical. Less intervention is necessary if limb use and ROM are progressing well and the pain response to manipulation is only mild, because many articular fractures are susceptible to failure and difficult to repair.

Spinal Cord Trauma

Unfortunately, neoplasia and infectious/inflammatory processes are a common cause of spinal cord dysfunction in cats (**Fig. 11**) and are often not amenable to rehabilitation. Intervertebral disk herniation is rare in cats, and traumatic spinal luxations and fractures are more common causes of acute spinal cord injury.[17] Postoperative nursing care is essential and the same as in dogs, with the exception of the unique temperament and special handling techniques characteristic of cats.[18]

Cruciate Ligament Injury

Cats are subject to cruciate ligament injury, but in contrast to dogs, cruciate ligament injury occurs primarily due to trauma.[13] As with spinal cord injuries, treatment and rehabilitation are similar to that in dogs. Of particular note in cats, they will commonly use their affected limb more readily postoperatively in comparison with dogs of similar size. Thus, it is very important to stress exercise restriction with particular focus on removing objects that the cat could jump on to. Stability of the joint, consistent weight-bearing, and maintenance of stifle extension are the main targets of immediate postoperative rehabilitation (first 3 weeks after surgery). Building muscle mass and strength are more important in the mid to late phases (3–6 weeks after surgery), once the stifle is stable.

REFERENCES

1. Lascelles BD, Dong YH, Marcellin-Little DJ, et al. Relationship of orthopedic examination, goniometric measurements, and radiographic signs of degenerative joint disease in cats. BMC Vet Res 2012;8:10.

2. Lascelles BD, Henry JB 3rd, Brown J, et al. Cross-sectional study of the prevalence of radiographic degenerative joint disease in domesticated cats. Vet Surg 2010;39:535–44.

3. Bennett D, Morton C. A study of owner observed behavioural and lifestyle changes in cats with musculoskeletal disease before and after analgesic therapy. J Feline Med Surg 2009;11:997–1004.

4. Jaeger GH, Marcellin-Little DJ, Depuy V, et al. Validity of goniometric joint measurements in cats. Am J Vet Res 2007;68:822–6.

5. Furlan AD, Imamura M, Dryden T, et al. Massage for low back pain: an updated systematic review within the framework of the Cochrane Back Review Group. Spine (Phila Pa 1976) 2009;34:1669–84.

6. Bockstahler B, Levine D, Millis D. Essential facts of physiotherapy in dogs and cats. 1st edition. Babenhausen (Germany): Be Vet Verlag; 2004.

7. Levine D, Millis DL, Mynatt T. Effects of 3.3-MHz ultrasound on caudal thigh muscle temperature in dogs. Vet Surg 2001;30:170–4.

8. Steiss JE, Adams CC. Effect of coat on rate of temperature increase in muscle during ultrasound treatment of dogs. Am J Vet Res 1999;60:76–80.

9. Steiss JE, Levine D. Physical agent modalities. Vet Clin North Am Small Anim Pract 2005;35:1317–33, viii.

10. Levine D, Bockstahler B. Electrical stimulation. In: Millis D, Levine D, editors. Canine rehabilitation and physical therapy. 2nd edition. Philadelphia: Saunders; 2014. p. 342–58.

11. Weigel J, Millis D. Therapeutic exercises and manual therapy. In: Millis D, Levine D, editors. Canine rehabilitation and physical therapy. 2nd edition. Philadelphia: Saunders; 2014. p. 401–542.

12. Welches CD, Scavelli TD. Transarticular pinning to repair luxation of the stifle joint in dogs and cats: a retrospective study of 10 cases. J Am Anim Hosp Assoc 1990;26:207–14.

13. McLaughlin RM. Surgical diseases of the feline stifle joint. Vet Clin North Am Small Anim Pract 2002;32:963–82.

14. Jaeger GH, Wosar MA, Marcellin-Little DJ, et al. Use of hinged transarticular external fixation for adjunctive joint stabilization in dogs and cats: 14 cases (1999-2003). J Am Vet Med Assoc 2005;227:586–91.

15. Taylor J, Tangner CH. Acquired muscle contractures in the dog and cat. A review of the literature and case report. Vet Comp Orthop Traumatol 2007;20:79–85.

16. Fries CL, Binnington AG, Cockshutt JR. Quadriceps contracture in four cats; a complication of internal fixation of femoral fractures. Vet Comp Orthop Traumatol 1988;2:91–6.

17. Salih F, Palus V, Cherubini GB. Acute spinal cord injury in the cat: causes, treatment and prognosis. J Feline Med Surg 2011;13:850–62.

18. Bockstahler B, Levine D. Physical therapy and rehabilitation. In: Norsworthy GD, Fooshee Grace S, Crystal MA, et al, editors. The feline patient. 4th edition. Ames (IA): Wiley-Blackwell; 2011. p. 687–90.

Index

Note: Page numbers of article titles are in **boldface** type.

Vet Clin Small Anim 45 (2015) 203–215
http://dx.doi.org/10.1016/S0195-5616(14)00163-6
0195-5616/15/$ – see front matter © 2015 Elsevier Inc. All rights reserved.

vetsmall.theclinics.com

Moving?

Make sure your subscription moves with you!

To notify us of your new address, find your **Clinics Account Number** (located on your mailing label above your name), and contact customer service at:

Email: journalscustomerservice-usa@elsevier.com

800-654-2452 (subscribers in the U.S. & Canada)
314-447-8871 (subscribers outside of the U.S. & Canada)

Fax number: 314-447-8029

Elsevier Health Sciences Division
Subscription Customer Service
3251 Riverport Lane
Maryland Heights, MO 63043

*To ensure uninterrupted delivery of your subscription, please notify us at least 4 weeks in advance of move.

Printed and bound by CPI Group (UK) Ltd, Croydon, CR0 4YY

18/10/2024

01775920-0001